BEHAVIOR MODIFICATION
AND THE NURSING PROCESS

BEHAVIOR MODIFICATION
AND THE NURSING PROCESS

ROSEMARIAN BERNI, R.N., M.N.

Assistant Professor, Physical Medicine and Rehabilitation,
University of Washington School of Medicine;
Adjunct Assistant Professor, Physiological Nursing,
University of Washington School of Nursing, Seattle, Washington

WILBERT E. FORDYCE, Ph.D.

Professor of Psychology,
Department of Rehabilitation Medicine and Pain Clinic,
University Hospital, University of Washington
School of Medicine, Seattle, Washington

SECOND EDITION

6 7 6 9

THE C. V. MOSBY COMPANY

SAINT LOUIS   1977

SECOND EDITION

Copyright © 1977 by The C. V. Mosby Company

Previous edition copyrighted 1973

Printed in the United States of America

Distributed in Great Britain by Henry Kimpton, London

The C. V. Mosby Company
11830 Westline Industrial Drive, St. Louis, Missouri 63141

Library of Congress Cataloging in Publication Data

Berni, Rosemarian, 1925-
   Behavior modification and the nursing process.

   Bibliography: p.
   1. Nursing—Psychological aspects.   2. Behavior
modification.   I. Fordyce, Wilbert Evans, 1923-   joint
author. II. Title.
RT86.B43   1977   610.73′01′9   76-57775
ISBN 0-8016-0656-X

VH/VH/VH   9   8   7   6   5   4   3   2   1

TO THE PATIENT

PREFACE

This revision of the book first published in 1973 reflects the experience and the feedback of readers of the earlier edition. The basic structure of the book remains the same. The changes are made mainly to clarify the use of behavioral methods by restating some points and by additional examples. New case examples illustrate kinds of patient care problems that lend themselves to these methods and provide details as to how to proceed. In addition, an expanded set of study examples at the end of several chapters should help to firm up the rudiments of the methods as the reader proceeds from one step to the next.

Since roughly the late 1950s, there has been virtually a revolution in the conceptualization of the nature of the problems people bring to human service and health care settings. More to the point, the newer conceptualizations have led to newer methods for helping people. The work of B. F. Skinner and a host of others, first in the laboratory with experimental animals and then in an ever-increasing range of human service settings, has demonstrated that the technology of behavior modification can help us to cope with many human performance problems that previously could not be dealt with rapidly if at all. Initially, these behavioral methods were applied mainly in the classroom, in child-rearing settings, and with the institutionalized mentally retarded or mentally ill. In more recent years, behavioral methods have begun to be applied in health care. This is the first book to set forth how behavioral methods can be applied "on line" in health care settings by nurses and other health care professionals in medical settings.

The key word is behavior. The process is behavior analysis. Other terms, such as operant conditioning, behavior modification, and contingency management, may also be used, and they mean about the same thing. This book seeks to acquaint nursing personnel and others working in the health care field with the rudiments of behavioral analysis and with procedures and principles to follow in applying behavioral analysis to a range of problems in their daily work.

Since 1964 we have been working with behavioral methods in health care settings. We have been testing the methods with a wide range of patient management problems. We have been teaching others how to use them. We have been involved also in the process of getting their use established in settings unacquainted with or non-responsive to their use. We share these objectives in presenting this book to you: to describe a tool by which nurses can help their patients; to describe some methods by which the patient can help himself; to suggest a vehicle by which the family can understand and support the patient's goals and simultaneously support the nurse's efforts toward those goals; to identify some approaches for helping staff to modify patient management techniques; to introduce a method by which all staff can actively participate in the patient management process; and to describe ways by which procedural steps can be made clear, specific, and immediately relevant to the patient's problems.

Human behavior is far too complex to permit a short book such as this one to provide all the answers to the daily problems encountered in the helping professions. The complex problems encountered in illness and disease and in the complicated subsociety of the health care system, with the multiplicity of professions and people involved in the patient's care, do not permit a brief book to provide magic formulas for success. What we think we can do is describe an approach to patient management problems that will outline practical techniques for helping your patients and for making your work both easier and more rewarding. This book will not solve all of your work problems. If it does not show you some immediately applicable methods to improve patient progress toward a variety of performance goals, we hope you reread it because the methods are there for the using.

This is a methods book. It seeks to provide nursing and other health care personnel with methods for accomplishing some of the patient care tasks with which they are confronted and for coping with some of the knotty or frustrating patient care problems that often arise. No change in patient goals or objectives is presented here, and no change is proposed in the basic philosophy of patient care and human services. Relating with patients in a meaningful way continues to be at the core of effective services. We do, however, have some suggestions to make about methods that may make exercise of basic treatment philosophies easier and more productive.

This book focuses on the central and predominant mode of behavioral methods: contingency management, or operant conditioning. This revised edition has added a number of demonstration problems and examples to help clarify further the application of these methods in health care settings.

If you, the reader, try to use these methods you will be trying to change patient behavior. You will also be trying to change colleague behavior. It is well to remember that behavior is behavior, whether it be that of a patient or a nurse. The most basic of all premises underlying the patient management methods set forth in this book is that behavior is influenced by consequences. The premise really goes beyond that for it is also usually true that behavior is not likely to change unless the immediate consequences to that behavior also change. It is to be expected, then, that what your patients do and what your colleagues do *both* will be influenced considerably by consequences of their behavior. As we note in more detail in Chapter 3, when you observe some behavior going on you can profitably assume it is being reinforced. That is true of nurses as well as patients. It follows that, if you try to change your colleagues' methods of doing things, you need to be concerned with what reinforcers are influencing their current behavior and what reinforcers will influence the new behaviors you are interested in getting them to use.

Teachers and directors of inservice training programs, among others, have long observed that showing "students" a new and different way of doing things is not by itself likely to bring about much change. That is often the case even where what is taught would appear to offer real advantages to the user. Sometimes it goes even beyond that. When a new method is introduced it may be greeted by resentment, passive resistance, or even open hostility. It is beyond the scope of these introductory remarks to go into all of the reasons why that happens. We shall content ourselves at this point with observing that patience is needed to bring about change. What is also needed is thoughtful consideration of the importance of helping your colleagues to receive much reinforcing encouragement during their early attempts at trying out these methods until their experience is sufficient that the even more durable reinforcers of successes with previously aggravating problems become clear and begin to occur.

Chapters 1 through 4 describe the analysis of behavior; Chapters 5 through 9 emphasize the reinforcement of behavior; and Chapters 10 through 14 involve system management, ethical issues, and future trends. All of the chapters are programmed to offer an assistive tool to nurse practitioners as they help their patients maintain or acquire functional progress, self-directiveness, and personal dignity.

We wish to extend our warmest appreciation to professional colleagues in the treatment programs of the Department of Rehabilitation Medicine, University of Washington Hospital, whose support rendered this work prossible.

Rosemarian Berni
Wilbert E. Fordyce

CONTENTS

1
INCREASING A BEHAVIOR

STATEMENT OF THE PROBLEM BY EXAMPLE

Mary, 62 years of age, was weak. She had been very ill. She had had a resection of the left femoral head and neck because of infection. After the operation she had hyponatremia, a myocardial infarction, acute tubular necrosis, and anemia. Three weeks after her heart attack, she was transferred to rehabilitation for ambulation training and for developing enough self-care skills to live independently. She learned and gained strength rapidly. However, despite her demonstrated skills at transferring from her bed, she routinely requested the bedpan instead of transferring to her bedside commode. In that sense she behaved in a way suggesting dependency on her nurse. It was important to establish use of the commode in order for her to live independently.

The problem facing the nurses was the very practical and real one of how to get Mary to use the commode instead of the bedpan. Instruction was tried but failed. Mary was urged to use the commode, and the importance of learning and practicing the use of it was emphasized. That also failed. We might have said that her dependency needs were too strong to relinquish that extra bit of help and attention from her nurses or that she was unmotivated to get better.

ANALYSIS OF BEHAVIOR

Let us consider another way of looking at her problem, follow a course of action it suggests, and observe the results. Let us look at

Mary's problem in behavioral terms. We think that the best way to proceed with understanding the behavioral approach is first to fix our eyes clearly on the target. What we are trying to do is help the patient, help her to be able to do things more or better than would be true if we did not work with her. Notice that we did not say "help her to be better." We said "help her to be able to do things more or better." If a patient can do more things or do them better, she will be better. The reverse is not always true. That is, a patient may feel better, at least for brief intervals, if she cannot do things and does not do them, and instead has them done for her. We may make our patient feel better by helping her, but that does not necessarily advance her treatment—it only makes her feel better. Helping Mary by bringing her the bedpan when she requested it might have made her feel better, but it would not have helped her be able to live independently. Helping patients feel better is very worthwhile, but it is not the goal of treatment. The goal of treatment is to help the patient to be able to do things. Over the long run, the more she can do the more she will be able to feel better.

In behavioral terms, Mary's problem was that she should have used the commode more and the bedpan less. Stated another way, the goal of treatment in that particular part of Mary's situation was to increase commode-using behavior and decrease bedpan-using behavior. To increase a behavior—that is, to make it occur more often —we need to do something about what happens *immediately after* the behavior occurs. What follows a behavior is a consequence. To increase the rate of a behavior, we need to do something about the immediate consequence of that behavior. When a bit of behavior is followed by a favorable or positive consequence (known also as a positive reinforcer), that behavior tends to occur more often or more consistently. To get Mary to use the commode more, we needed to be sure that use of the commode was followed immediately by a favorable consequence, or positive reinforcer. Mary's nurses noted that Mary very much enjoyed talking with them. They could see that their attention to or social interaction with Mary had positive value to her. Therefore, they programmed themselves to let their value to Mary be put to work to help Mary with her problem. Their basic strategy about selection of reinforcers was to draw on things in which they knew the patient had a positive interest. This illustrates a basic principle that will be discussed in Chapter 5 when the topic of reinforcers and their selection will receive detailed attention. Specifically, when Mary asked for the commode, it was provided, and one of the nursing personnel would stay with her to chat for awhile. In contrast, when Mary asked for the bedpan, it was given freely, but the nurse left rather than staying to chat. Within a few days, Mary used only the commode. She continued to do so for the rest of her hospitalization, even though her nurses discontinued the special reinforcement arrangement after Mary began using the commode consistently.

The program used by the nurses to help Mary illustrates several major points about the use of patient management techniques based on behavioral principles. A most important point is to note that the methods used followed good nursing techniques and emphasized the important role nurses play in the lives of their patients. We refer to the nursing relationship. Because the nurses had established a working relationship with Mary, because they had been able to relate and communicate with her, they were able to help. Had they ignored her or behaved toward her in such a way that she would feel isolated or rejected, the program they used would likely have had little effect. The relationship with the patient is essential to good nursing care in any chronic illness setting. That is no less true of behavioral approaches than of other methods of trying to help our patients.

The program with Mary illustrates some other basic points about behavioral systems. Notice that the program used did not attempt to change some of Mary's attitudes or feelings (such as dependency and lack of motivation). The program aimed directly at what Mary was doing, her behavior. The nurses did not, for example, try to motivate Mary further to use the commode. That had already been tried without success. They did not try to change her attitudes about dependency on nurses. They helped Mary to change her behavior.

In pinpointing Mary's problem in behavioral terms, we noted that she needed to increase use of the commode and decrease use of the bedpan. That brings us to the next point. Analysis of a patient management problem in behavioral terms can usually narrow the problem down to one of three possibilities. Either the patient is not doing enough of something (he or she needs to increase a behavior) or is doing too much of something (he or she needs to decrease a behavior). If the problem can be defined in behavioral terms and it is not one of these possibilities, the only other possibility is that the patient needs to do something and does not know how to do it. We will deal with that possibility later when we discuss shaping.

We suggest that when nursing personnel analyze patient management problems in behavioral terms, they can often come up with practical and sometimes quite simple solutions. This book is directed toward illustrating the use of these behavioral analysis methods in everyday problems of nursing care. Our objective is to equip nursing personnel with skills in the use of these methods sufficient to permit them to deal effectively with many patient care problems.

The analysis of Mary's problem in behavioral terms led to the decision to try to increase a particular behavior (use of commode) by letting it be followed immediately by a favorable consequence or positive reinforcer: socializing with her nurse. Instead of trying to change an attitude or feeling so that behavior would change, her nurses helped her by putting their attention to work in a systematic way. Imagine what would have happened if her nurses chatted freely with her whenever their schedule permitted them to do so, no matter what Mary was doing. They might have had a nice relationship with her, but they quite likely would have failed to help her shift from using a bedpan to using a commode.

Behavior is action. Behavior is something people do. When you as a nurse try to help a patient begin to do more of something he or she needs to do more of (as in Mary's case, use the commode), you are asking your patient to change behavior. You are not asking your patient to change motivation or attitudes, but to change what he or she actually does. We are so ingrained with the idea that one must understand a person's motivations in order to know what he or she is going to do that it is very difficult to step back and take another look at the situation. Perhaps it will help if you can recognize that using concepts about a person's underlying motivation is only one of a number of possible ways of going about the business of understanding and helping to change behavior. It is not true that one must understand a person's motivation in order to predict what the person is going to do. It is only true that trying to understand underlying motivations is one of a number of possible ways of trying to understand and of being capable of changing what a person does.

Notice something else about this matter. Even if you use the concept of motivation as a way of trying to organize your thoughts about patients so that you can be in a better position to help them, you still must come back to what they do, their behavior. If, as in Mary's case, commode use goes up, you can, if you wish, choose to conclude that Mary's motivation changed. Suppose the program failed and Mary continued to use the bedpan just as she had at the outset. You might conclude that her motivation had remained unchanged. Notice, however, that whether you succeeded or failed, your conclusions were based on what Mary did; that is, she increased or decreased use of the bedpan or commode. Your conclusions were based on her behavior. If you continued to use the concept of motivation, it was only as an after-the-fact way of rationalizing what happened. What Mary did was to use the bedpan or commode. What you did was to try to explain or rationalize Mary's behavior. By bringing in the concept of motivation, you changed nothing.

Example—behavior change, not motivation

Consider another example to illustrate further that it is usually what a patient does, his behavior, that is the real concern for us. Mrs. L was paraplegic, paralyzed from the waist down. Among other problems, she had a loss of bowel and bladder control. People in such a plight must drink enough fluids to result in a daily bladder output level of approximately 3,000 ml in order to maintain kidney function and avoid bladder infections. Mrs. L had been in the hospital several months. She had rather consistently failed to drink the 4,000 ml of fluid each day that her doctor felt was essential to her well-being. In her quiet, withdrawn way, she would listen docilely to repeated instructions and exhortations regarding the importance of drinking 4,000 ml per day. She usually would express chagrin at her failure to perform and voice promises to do better. In fact, daily records of fluid intake showed a definite, though gradual, downward trend to her fluid intake.

There were a number of possible explanations to account for Mrs. L's behavior. We might have inferred that she was unmotivated to get better, perhaps that she felt safer in the hospital and so behaved in ways designed to keep her in the hospital. We might have inferred that she was passive-aggressive; that is, superficially cooperative but subtly resistant and rebellious and therefore motivated to resist authority. We might have concluded she was either too depressed to perform (except that her general manner hardly suggested depression) or that she was trying to destroy herself—perhaps because the prospect of being paraplegic the rest of her life was intolerable or because she felt guilt over either her accident or the burden that she felt she was placing on her family. Any one or a combination of these possibilities was plausible in light of what she was actually doing: drinking only about 1,200 to 1,400 ml per day.

Mrs. L's treatment team chose not to focus on what her underlying motivations might be. They chose to try to change the behavior that clearly needed changing: daily fluid intake. Instead of trying to develop approaches aimed at modifying an inferred underlying motivation or attitude, they took direct aim at her behavior. They asked themselves the question, "What are the immediate consequences when Mrs. L drinks fluids?" The answer was that there were no immediate consequences—or at any rate no consistent immediate consequences.

Such consequences that did occur usually came the morning after a day of inadequate fluid intake, when her physician and her nurse, noting the charted amount of fluid output, reminded her or exhorted her to better effort. Note two things there. First, what they wanted her to do more of was to drink fluids. If she drank more fluids, there would be more output. In this case, you cannot increase output without increasing input. Yet, initially they had not been focusing on the behavior that needed to change, fluid intake. Second, the consequences that they were delivering were delayed until the next day, several hours after the behavior they needed to change: drinking.

Upon reflection, the team changed its approach. They bypassed attitudes and motivations and focused on behavior: the actions of Mrs. L; namely, drinking. They provided her with a small clipboard to which was fixed a sheet of paper laid out on an hourly schedule, with columns in which how much she drank could be recorded each time she took in fluids and with columns in which cumulative totals could be recorded. As a reminder to the staff, a column was also provided that the staff could initial to indicate they had checked the totals and had responded to her performance with their attention. Mrs. L kept her clipboard with her as she moved from place to place in her wheelchair. Whenever she approached, nurses and therapists, seeing the clipboard, were reminded to offer her fluids. When she accepted, they were able to respond immediately to her drinking behavior. Under the impact of these systematic responses to her drinking behavior, Mrs. L increased her fluid intake rate rapidly to well above the target level of 4,000 ml per day.

Did her motivation, her attitudes, her possible passive-aggressive traits, her possible depression, or guilt change? Perhaps. One thing is sure, her behavior changed. Moreover, after a few weeks, the fluid intake habit was well established and persisted without further use of the clipboard.

What Mrs. L needed was to change her drinking behavior. Her program took direct aim at that and not at some other kind of target, such as attitude or mood or motivation.

PRACTICE PROBLEMS

The focus on behavior or actions and not on indirect matters, such as feelings, motivations, or attitudes, is of essential importance to behavior modification. If this first and very major point is not well understood, what follows in this book will not be well understood. Some thought about the following examples should be of further help.

1. A depressed patient refuses to get out of bed to practice an important exercise, walking. What is the behavior to be changed?
   a. Depression? No, that is a feeling or mood state, not behavior.
   b. Motivation? No, that is a feeling or mood state, not behavior.
   c. Resistance? No, that is not specific enough.
   d. Walking? Yes, that is what needs to be increased.
2. An angry, sullen patient needles her nurses by calling them every few minutes. What is the behavior to be changed?
   a. Anger? No, that is not a behavior.
   b. Negativism? No, that is not a behavior.
   c. Pushing the call button? Yes, that is the behavior that needs to be reduced in frequency.
3. An elderly, moderately senile patient with occasional memory lapses forgets to zip closed his trousers and walks about the ward exposing himself. What is the behavior to be changed?
   a. Memory loss? No, that is not a specific behavior.
   b. Regression? No, that is not a specific behavior.
   c. Trouser zipping? Yes, that is what should be increased.
4. A patient resists taking medications. He always argues with his nurse before smallowing his medications. What is the behavior to be changed?
   a. Negativism? No, that is not a behavior.
   b. Lack of motivation to get better? No, that is not a behavior.
   c. Taking medications? No, he is already doing that.
   d. Arguing with his nurse? Yes, that is what should be decreased.

SUMMARY

1. Behavior is action. Behavior is something a person does.
2. Behavior may be increased (helped to occur more often) by following the behavior with a favorable consequence or positive reinforcer.

2
DECREASING A BEHAVIOR

STATEMENT OF THE PROBLEM

In the preceding chapter we talked about increasing a behavior that had too low a rate. In this chapter we consider how to decrease a behavior that occurs too often.

Let us return once again to the case of Mary. We observed earlier that Mary's problem could be analyzed into either increasing a behavior (use of commode) or decreasing a behavior (use of bedpan). The choice was made in that case to attempt to increase commode-using behavior by following that behavior with a positive reinforcer: socializing with her nurse. We also noted that the special socializing with her nurse occurred only when Mary used the commode and not just at any time. That brings us to the next point.

We have said that a behavior may be increased by arranging to follow it promptly with positive reinforcement. It can now be added that the frequency of a behavior may be reduced by withdrawing the positive reinforcement it has been receiving. When a behavior fails to lead to positive reinforcement, it begins to diminish in frequency or strength. For example, in Mary's case her nurses were careful not to stay to socialize with her when she requested the bedpan. Had they stayed, they risked providing positive reinforcement in the form of their presence and attention. The effect likely would have been to help maintain the very behavior they were trying to help Mary reduce; namely, use of bedpan.

The principle here is the logical extention of the point of Chapter 1. If a behavior is positively reinforced, it tends to strengthen or increase. In the same vein, if a behavior is not positively reinforced, it will tend to diminish and eventually disappear. The process is known as *extinction*.

There are several points to be made about extinction, or helping a person to reduce the rate of a behavior. Perhaps most important is that there are two basic ways of going about it. One is to withdraw reinforcement from the behavior to be reduced. The second is to attach effective reinforcement to the alternative behavior; that is, to effectively reinforce the behavior the patient needs to be doing *instead* of the behavior you are trying to help him or her to reduce. These two approaches may be used separately or together. We can use the example of Mary again to illustrate. The problem with Mary might be analyzed as one in which she is either helped to reduce use of the bedpan *or* helped to increase use of the commode. A program to bring about that behavior change might focus on withdrawing reinforcement to use of the bedpan *or* on attaching effective reinforcement to the desirable alterative, use of the commode, or both.

How does one decide which way to go: to withdraw reinforcement and strive for extinction or to focus on reinforcing the more desired alternative behavior? The choice is usually fairly easy to make. The guiding principles are:

1. It is nearly always easier to accelerate or increase a behavior with positive reinforcement than it is to decelerate or decrease a behavior by extinction.
2. If a person is to stop doing something, he or she needs something else to do in its place.
3. In order for the behavior change to occur, the "old" behavior must no longer receive effective reinforcement and the "new" behavior must receive effective reinforcement.

We can return to Mary's case to illustrate further the use of these principles. Mary's nurses might have decided simply to withdraw their attention from use of the bedpan in the hope of relying on extinction to solve the problem. That would have been an unwise choice, in relation to the principles listed above. It is not enough to expect someone not to do something. The person must have an alternative. In Mary's case, the commode is the logical alternative but in order to be more sure she would come to use it, that choice needs some reinforcement.

As has been seen, the *nurses* shifted the positive reinforcers represented by their attention. They withdrew the reinforcement from the "old" or bedpan behavior, and they attached it to the "new" or commode behavior.

This brings us to another point about extinction and why it is more difficult to bring about than increasing an alternative behavior. Usually our behavior is supported by a complex multiplicity of reinforcement. A behavior change process that seeks to withdraw reinforcement from a behavior will often find that only some of the reinforcement has been withdrawn. Other sources or kinds of reinforcement continue to be available to help support continuation of the behavior to be reduced. Thus relying solely on the extinction process is inherently at some risk because one is unlikely to be able to end totally a prevailing reinforcement pattern. This is one major reason why helping a person to develop an alternative behavior that is to be reinforced is easier than striving only to end reinforcement to the old behavior. In Mary's case use of the bedpan was probably being sustained or reinforced in several ways prior to the start of the behavior change process. For example, considering her disability, it was probably less arduous to use the bedpan than to make a body transfer from the bed to a commode. That "naturally occurring" reinforcement would continue even if nurse attention was withdrawn to the bedpan behavior. The change the nurses instituted programmed a reinforcement, their attention, to compete with the naturally occurring reinforcement to the old behavior. When the bedpan was requested and used, they left. When the commode was requested and used, in the early phases of the change process, they stayed to provide the support of their social responsiveness to the strengthening of the new and alternative behavior.

It should be remembered that withdrawal of reinforcement from a behavior is rarely sufficient in itself to help a person to change. Additional reinforcers may continue in the picture to help maintain the behavior that one is trying to extinguish. Additionally, the person may not have an effective and effectively reinforced behavior to change *to*. In short, it is true that a behavior will tend to diminish and even disappear totally if reinforcement is withdrawn. But, in the practical case, that kind of change can better be brought about by focusing on *both* withdrawing reinforcement to the "old" and attaching reinforcement to the "new."

Examples—decrease a behavior

The case of Mr. B illustrates these points further. Mr. B was in his mid-40's. He had a chronic pain problem for which he had had approximately a dozen operations that had not reduced or eliminated his pain. The last several operations had involved cutting nerve fibers in an attempt to reduce his pain. One of those cordotomies had left him with a partial loss of bladder control, so that he would occasionally have a minor bladder accident if he let his bladder become too full. He also experienced a sense of urgency to empty his bladder at frequent intervals. The result was that his activities during the day and his sleep at night were interrupted by the feeling that he needed to empty his bladder. Typically, he would arise three to four times during the night to go to the bathroom. In the daytime it was even more frequent: approximately every 30 to 45 minutes. Mr. B had many problems, but we are concerned here only with the matter of bladder frequency. It was a problem because it interrupted his sleep, thereby increasing his fatigue and aggravating his pain, and because it disrupted daytime activities that could have served to distract him from pain.

Mr. B's nurses analyzed his bladder frequency problem in behavioral terms. The behavior they wanted to change was to decrease the frequency of emptying his bladder, but without decreasing that frequency so much that his bladder would become overly distended and bladder accidents would occur. His physicians judged that his daily consumption of fluids was such that emptying his bladder twice a day at appropriately dispersed intervals would meet his needs adequately. The treatment plan selected was to decrease bladder-draining frequency by attaching positive reinforcers to a replacement behavior: "bladder-saving" behavior. So far as could be judged, the positive reinforcers Mr. B had been receiving for frequent emptying of his bladder was that he remained dry. There was very little that could be done to withdraw that reinforcer from his too frequent emptying behavior—nor would one want to. What could be done, however, was to attach other, positive reinforcers to bladder-saving behavior and to organize the program in such a way that he would also remain dry. That would let the positive reinforcement of dryness, as well, be attached to the new behavior.

A program to help Mr. B reduce bladder frequency had an advantage. The bladder frequency behavior was not inherently and directly reinforcing. It was being maintained out of fear of the consequences were he to act differently. Stated another way, he didn't have an acceptable alternative. Therefore, the problem basically was one of reducing one behavior by helping him to find another, while being sure that other behavior received ample positive reinforcement during its developmental stages.

The treatment plan that the nurses followed was simple to carry

out. First they explained the whole program to Mr. B; what they proposed to do and how they proposed to do it. He agreed to participate.
His fluid intake was fairly constant. For the next several days they
had him record on a diary form when he emptied his bladder. (How
can you know whether any treatment program has helped change
behavior if you do not know how much the behavior is occurring in
the first place?) They also had him drain his bladder into a beaker
from which output measures could be obtained at two preselected
times of day: approximately 7:30 AM and 10:00 PM. Those times
were selected because they were appropriately dispersed to avoid excessive accumulations of urine and because those times helped minimize interference in daily activities or sleep. After a few days of recording, his nurses knew about how much he typically produced at
the two target times. They then set quotas for him to reach at those
times. The quotas started at his own average output and were increased by 20 ml each day. They talked with Mr. B and asked him
to select rewards (positive reinforcers) that he could win by meeting
his quotas. His choices were a cocktail before dinner (he provided
his own liquor supply) if he met the morning quota and a telephone
call if he met the evening quota. If he failed to meet a quota, he did
not receive his reinforcement. The increases in successfully met quotas
are shown in Figure 1.

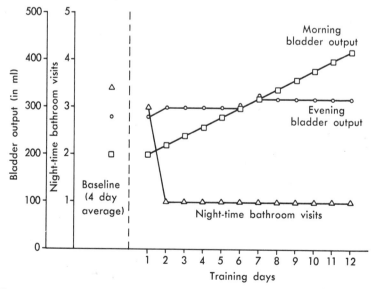

Figure 1. Decreased nocturnal awakening with bladder urgency by reinforcement.

What about all of the other times that he emptied his bladder each day and night? These were ignored. He received no attention from his nurses nor any urging from them to try not to go to the bathroom as frequently. All of the reinforcers programmed with Mr. B were directed at increasing the amount he could produce at the target times. He could not produce more if he did not save. In short, his nurses tried to decrease a behavior by positively reinforcing a replacement behavior. The third night after the reinforcement program began, Mr. B slept through the night. Thereafter for the five weeks that he was under observation, he never had to arise at night to empty his bladder, nor did he have bladder accidents. The frequency of daytime bladder emptying dropped markedly, though not to zero. When an adequate outcome had been reached, quotas were leveled off and the special reinforcements were terminated, without changing his performance. Ten months later, he reported continuing success without further need for a special incentive program.

When considering behaviors to be decreased, we must recognize that if a behavior is occurring with some frequency, either it is being directly reinforced or alternative behaviors are not being reinforced and perhaps are even being punished. The example of young Bert illustrates this point further. Bert presented the kind of problem that one might find in a child care setting. Bert was 4½ years old. His problem was that he messed his pants several times a day and, of course, that he failed to make his deposits in the toilet more than very occasionally. His parents and his day care nurse (both of his parents worked during the day) had tried a variety of approaches ranging from bribery and punishment to therapy by a child psychiatrist, all without success.

Bert's parents were asked first to keep a record for one week when he was noted to have messy pants and to indicate exactly what they did. The pattern quickly emerged. Interestingly enough, Bert did not seem to be upset at spending the day in the day care setting, as one might have expected. So far as could be judged, this setting, involving only two other children of nearly the same age, was rather stimulating and enjoyable to him. His accidents seemed to be about equally distributed between those at home (early morning and evenings) and those at the day care center. The sequence was that, when his messy pants were detected, he was taken to the bathroom, cleaned up, and (sometimes) put on the toilet for awhile before being dressed and returned to whatever activities were going on. When these accidents occurred, the adults in the situation made much over it. He was sometimes criticized, sometimes exhorted to use the toilet, and sometimes threatened with loss of some privilege or another. When he did not have accidents, he received reasonable amount of attention, though certainly not a rich amount.

His parents were instructed in the idea that their attention and responsiveness was quite possibly going too much toward a behavior they really wanted to decrease and not enough to the behavior they wanted to increase: using the toilet. Moreover, relationships between Bert and his parents—and his day care nurses—were becoming increasingly strained so that the quality of attention was more and more abrasive. The next step was to withdraw attention as a systematic consequence to accident behavior and to attach that consequence to the behavior to be increased, using the toilet. Specifically, the three adults working with Bert were instructed to be noncommittal to accidents. They would say nothing more than to offer to take him to the bathroom to help him clean up. In carrying out this chore, they would carry on an absolute minimum of conversation with him and strive to maintain a neutral, noncommittal manner. They were also to instruct Bert that each time he used the toilet appropriately, he would receive praise and a gold star charted plainly where Bert and his parents could see it. As the program progressed, increasing numbers of gold stars earned special events, such as fishing with his father or playing catch.

The essence of the program with Bert was that attention was withdrawn from the behavior to be decreased (accidents) and attached to the behavior to be increased, using the toilet. Figure 2 shows the results. Notice from Figure 2 that when the reinforcer of attention was first withdrawn from the behavior to be decreased, it in fact increased. That is usually the case. When a reinforcer is withdrawn from a behavior, that behavior tends initially to increase before it begins to decrease.* In Bert's case, the third day after the new program was begun he had eight accidents, with the last one occurring in the middle of the living room 15 minutes before dinner guests arrived. Fortunately for Bert, his parents had the courage of lions. They held steady to the program, and all involved, including Bert, were rewarded by a steady reduction in the accident behavior. After a very few weeks, all special arrangements were dropped, and Bert carried on well by himself. Once established, effective toilet behavior provided many

---

*This point is illustrated when a smoker tries to quit smoking. The first few hours and days his rate of wanting to smoke actually increases before it begins to decrease. The same thing usually happens with the desire to eat when one starts a diet.

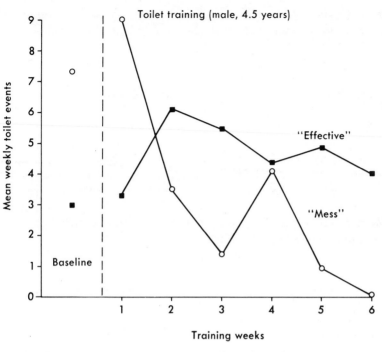

Figure 2. Decreased bowel accidents.

naturally occurring "payoffs" or reinforcers to Bert, so that his parents did not need to maintain for very long their special reinforcement efforts. This point receives more detailed discussion in Chapter 5 when reinforcement is considered.

SUMMARY

The major behavior change principles that we have dealt with so far are:

1. Behavior or actions are primary targets for nursing personnel in helping patients. What patients need is to be able to do things more or better, not to feel better.
2. Behavior may be changed by changing consequences or reinforcers.
3. Patient problems involving behavior change can usually be broken down into one of the following possibilities:
    a. A behavior is not occurring as often or as much as it needs to and should be increased. That problem should be changed by attaching positive reinforcers to the behavior.

b. A behavior is occurring more often than it should and needs to be decreased. That should be changed by withdrawing positive reinforcers to the behavior and attaching reinforcers to a more desirable replacement behavior.

Of the case examples thus far considered, all but one have relied on a combination of withdrawing reinforcement from one behavior and attaching reinforcement to another. The bedpan/commode problem with Mary, the fluid intake problem with Mrs. L, and the toilet training problem with Bert all strived to diminish social reinforcement (attention) to the old behavior and to attach that reinforcement to the new. In the case of Mr. B's bladder frequency problem, the choice was even simpler. He was simply helped to develop an alternative behavior.

4. Withdrawing reinforcers from a behavior is rarely sufficient in itself to bring about a behavior change.
   a. Some residual reinforcement is likely to continue.
   b. The person may not have an effective alternative behavior or that alternative behavior may not receive sufficient initial reinforcement to become established.
5. It is easier to increase or accelerate a behavior than to decrease or decelerate a behavior.
6. The preferred choice in helping a person to decrease a behavior is nearly always to focus primarily on helping to establish an alternative behavior by effective reinforcement, while attempting nonetheless to diminish reinforcement to the "old" behavior.

PRACTICE PROBLEMS

The careful analysis of behavior change problems is essential. One of the key issues is to be clear in your own mind whether the focus of the plan is to help a person decrease one behavior or to increase another or both. The following problems may help to clarify how to use the guiding principles.

1. A youngster consistently drops his coat and hat on the floor when entering the house. The mission is to get him to hang up the garments. The behavior is reinforced mainly in that it gives him quicker access to whatever he wanted to do upon entering the house. He doesn't have to take the time to go to the closet to hang up things. Moreover, hanging-up behavior receives only intermittent, and often quite delayed, praise from his mother. The question is whether one should focus on extinction of dropping behavior or on increasing of hanging-up behavior.
   a. *Extinction of dropping behavior:* This might be accomplished

by withdrawing the existing reinforcement that occurs when mother picks up after him and hangs the garments in the closet, but it does not seem likely. An additional step might be to put the garments where he could not reach them and to prohibit going outside without them. Thus the reinforcers available from outside play become contingent upon hanging up the garments. That is a possibility.

b. *Increasing hanging-up behavior:* This might be accomplished by attaching positive reinforcers to that behavior. For example, a chart with gold stars as reinforcers might be posted at an appropriate place, and hanging-up behavior would earn stars. Another approach would be to let TV time be earned by performance of various self-care and household chores, including hanging-up behavior.

It is probably simpler and more effective to focus on increasing the hanging-up behavior because the reinforcers can become more immediately available and are more readily controlled. The probably powerful reinforcer of TV time might serve as a very effective incentive.

2. A patient with chronic pain spends much of the day reclining. Once it is medically established that the patient is capable of and would benefit from greater activity, behavioral approaches might be considered.* Here we might consider that choice as being between withdrawing reinforcement for reclining behavior or attaching reinforcement to nonreclining behavior (e.g., walking, sitting).

a. *Reduction of reclining behavior:* Many pain patients receive extra attention of solicitousness from family and health care professionals if their problem is displayed by a variety of communications to those around them that pain is felt. One such behavior is to recline when otherwise one would be moving about. In the hospital setting or at home those working with the patient might be helped to reserve conversations for those occasions when the patient was dressed and out of bed. Attention is withdrawn from reclining.

b. *Increasing activity level:* Both attention or social responsiveness of those around the patient and rest may be used to reinforce gradually increasing amounts of walking and other exer-

*A detailed consideration of the use of behavioral concepts in relation to problems of chronic pain can be found in Fordyce, W.: *Behavioral Methods for Chronic Pain and Illness,* St. Louis, 1976, The C. V. Mosby Co., 236 pp.

cise. Examples of this are given in Chapter 5 in the discussion of rest as a reinforcer.

The choice here seems clearly to work on both "a" and "b"; that is, help to diminish attention for the sick or pain behaviors of excessive reclining and to increase the more healthful alternative of walking and exercise.

3. A patient yells and curses freely when working with the nurse, physical therapist, occupational therapist, or other health worker. The alternatives are to withdraw reinforcement to cursing or to reinforce work and/or conversation without cursing.

    a. *Decreasing cursing:* If the patient curses, leave, thus making your (the professional's) presence contingent upon noncursing. Stated another way, presence as a social reinforcer is withdrawn if the behavior to be reduced occurs. (Another illustration of this approach is given in Chapter 5.)

    b. *Increasing noncursing:* When the patient is working with you or is conversing with you without cursing, converse. If the patient curses, remain silent. Your conversing is now attached to the patient's noncursing behavior.

Since the reinforcer one is attempting to use here is the same for both approaches (i.e., attention), the approaches are but mirror images of each other. To use one is also to use the other. Moreover, both changes have to occur; that is, one must both withdraw conversation to one set of behaviors and attach it to the other. Attention or conversation becomes contingent. This point receives detailed attention in Chapter 5.

3
PINPOINTING THE TARGET

STATEMENT OF THE PROBLEM

As you go about analyzing patient management problems, you should try to identify as precisely as possible what behavior needs to be changed; that is, what behavior needs to be increased or decreased. This must be done precisely, not vaguely: for example, to set your goal or target as that of helping the patient to be able to take care of himself better is too vague and general. Precisely what is it that the patients needs to do more or less of? Precisely what behavior is to change? Let us examine another example to illustrate this point. Lori was a girl in her early teens who had sustained a head injury in an accident. Her head injury resulted in permanent brain damage that left her with, among other problems, memory difficulties and a tendency to be careless, a frequent pattern in many brain-injured patients. Those ways of behaving had not been at all like her prior to her injury, but they were now a major concern to her family and the rehabilitation team working with her. The problem with which we shall concern ourselves here is how to get Lori to do her ADLs (activities of daily living, such as bathing, dressing, combing her hair, brushing her teeth, and making her bed).

Examples—pinpointing behavior

Lori was able to use her hands and to walk with only mild impairment. She knew how to do each of her ADLs and she had the physical ability to do them. The problem was that she did not remember to do them consistently. Her nurse's first effort at helping Lori with this problem was to be sure that Lori knew how to do each of the tasks and that she knew she was expected to do them. That did not improve Lori's performance very much, and the little gain she made lasted only a day or two. Next, her nurse tried giving her more systematic reminders by posting a list of the ADLs beside her bed so that she could see what it was she was supposed to do. There was some improvement, but Lori's performance remained inconsistent. From the behavioral analysis point of view, we could say that her nurse had taken a first important step by moving from the vague general goal of doing self-care, or ADLs, to more precise specifying and listing of what it was that Lori was expected to do. The nurse had not yet, however, arranged systematic consequences to each of those behaviors. After consultation with her colleagues, she took that next step. She assigned one point to each of the five tasks that the team felt were important for Lori to perform. She then worked out a plan with Lori in which access to Lori's radio during the evening hours depended on the number of points Lori earned in the morning by doing her ADLs.* Each point earned provided her with 10 minutes of radio time. If she performed all five tasks, a bonus of unlimited radio time was awarded. Results are shown in Figure 3. This method illustrates use of a token or point system. Details about problems and methods for using token systems are discussed and illustrated in Chapter 6.

This approach had a number of advantages for Lori. By providing Lori with the list of ADLs, the nurse gave Lori an immediate reminder. At the same time, by putting a premium on complete performance, the nurse gave Lori an added reminder to check herself to be sure that everything was done. There was also, of course, the additional advantage that the method helped the nurse not to have to nag Lori, thereby making it much easier to maintain an effective and positive relationship with her.

Notice from Figure 3, as in the earlier examples, that Lori's nurse was careful first to count the rate of the behavior that was to be changed before she began the final effort to change the behavior.

---

*The important ethical and practical issues relating to patient consent and participation in these approaches are dealt with in Chapter 13. For now let us note that Lori was asked if she would use an incentive method—to which she readily agreed—and was asked to choose the incentive that her nurse would then program.

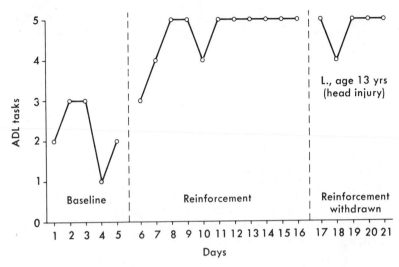

Figure 3. Increased ADL performance using a token system.

Establishing that baseline is of critical importance. Unless we know how much the behavior is occurring before trying to change it, we will not know whether the change efforts are having effect. Notice also that after several days of reinforcement, Lori's nurse withdrew the reinforcer of the use of radio (giving her unlimited access to it), and Lori's performance continued to hold up. Lori had been the one to mark the chart on the wall that recorded her ADL performance. She quite obviously took considerable pride in her performance. After the first day or two it is highly questionable whether the radio was any longer the critical reinforcer. Pride and sense of accomplishment probably had taken over. So when Lori s nurse, with Lori's consent of course, let the radio be accessible whether or not the ADLs had been done, it indicated that Lori had in fact taken over. More precisely stated, Lori's behavior had now come under control of naturally occurring reinforcers (Lori's pride), an important point that is dealt with in the chapter on generalization.

The major point in this example is that Lori's nurse quickly found out that when she formulated the target behavior in general terms (stated as "clean up yourself and your room" or "you should be neat and clean"), neither the patient nor the nurse could tell whether it was occurring well enough or not. In addition, when the target behavior was stated in general terms, it was not possible to arrange for specific reinforcement of specific behaviors.

Another brief example illustrates this important point further. Mr. J, who was in his 50's had been paraplegic for several years. He was a bachelor who had a lady friend who was a nurse (which, as we shall see, may or may not have been to his advantage). He had been hospitalized with a skin breakdown that had resulted from his not having been consistently careful in his skin care. He had been overly reliant on his nurse friend to help him with many aspects of his self-care program; for example, catheter irrigation and checking his skin. His friend's work schedule was such that she could not be relied upon to provide systematic assistance in self-care activities. His skin healed, and the date of discharge approached; but the team was still faced with the problem of helping him to establish an effective habit of self-care; that is of getting him to carry out his particular set of ADLs instead of relying on his girlfriend.

Mr. J's performance (or lack of it) could have been characterized as a motivational problem. Or, as with our first example, Mary, we might have said that he had careless attitudes, perhaps even that he had self-destructive impulses. Approached from the behavioral analysis viewpoint, the focus is on what it was he needed to do more or less of. However, even then, it is sometimes the case that the target behaviors get defined in too broad terms; for example, "he needs to do his ADLs." If his nurses had worked out with him some kind of reinforcement pattern whereby he would receive the reinforcers when he had done his ADLs the tasks would still not have been specific enough to permit precise programming of reinforcers. For example, if he did six of the nine things he needed to do, would he be reinforced or not? If he was reinforced for doing only part of the set of tasks, his nurses would have, in effect, reinforced him for some good and some bad (nonperformance) behavior. To do that would tend to perpetuate the problem, not solve it. Moreover, if the patient was not entirely sure just what he was to do, it would have been more difficult for him to perform, just as was true of Lori in the preceding example. If our efforts to help our patients change behavior are to be effective, we must be precise in specifying with them what it is that they need to do more or less of.

Mr. J's nurses worked out with him the list of ADL and self-care activities that it was important for him to do. They then worked out a contract with him (and his girlfriend) whereby performance of each task in the morning earned 10 minutes of visiting time with his nurse friend in the evening. Mr. J. reached the 100% level in performance of his ADLs. This is another illustration of use of a token or point system. The points served as a promise that reinforcement would be delivered at a later time, thereby bridging the time gap between behavior and reinforcement. Chapter 6 will deal with these methods in some detail.

PRACTICE PROBLEMS

For some more target practice, try the following examples.

1. A stroke patient prefers resting and sleeping on his back and thereby risks developing decubiti. What is the behavior to be changed?
   a. Bed mobility? No, that is too general.
   b. Reclining on the unaffected side? Yes, that is what he needs to increase.

2. A withdrawn and a somewhat depressed nursing home patient spends all day in bed instead of going to the dayroom or moving around for exercise. Joint contractures and decubiti are real hazards. What is the behavior to be changed?
   a. Withdrawal? No, that is too vague.
   b. Depression? No, that is too vague and a feeling, not a behavior.
   c. Walking? Yes, that is one thing he needs to increase.
   d. Playing checkers (in dayroom)? Yes, that is a behavior, which, if increased, means that walking (to get there) was increased and that time in bed has decreased.

3. A patient who has had a myocardial infarction so fears another attack that he refuses to cooperate in a graduated walking and exercise program, the limits of which have been carefully defined by his doctor. What is the behavior to be changed?
   a. Fear? No, that is not a specific behavior.
   b. Activity level? No, that is vague, not specific.
   c. Walking? Yes, that is a specific, observable and measurable behavior.

4. A recently disabled quadriplegic patient with some hand function is learning enough typing to permit him to replace lost writing ability. The patient, preoccupied with recent losses, sits at the typewriter table in Occupational Therapy and gazes out the window, lost in ruminative fantasy. What is the behavior to be changed?
   a. Decrease rumination or fantasy? No, that is not a behavior.
   b. Decrease depression? No, that is a feeling not a behavior.
   c. Increase acceptance of disability? No, that is too vague.
   d. Increase typing? Yes. That is a behavior, it is specific, and it leads to mastery of a task or function which itself can lead

to further reinforcement. That is how depression relating to onset of disability is overcome: reinforcement for and mastery of disability-appropriate behaviors.

5. A patient with painful joint contractures secondary to body burns is going through range-of-motion exercises but performance is repeatedly interrupted or limited by excessive pain. What is the behavior to be changed?

   a. Reduce pain? No, that is vague, unspecific, and not a behavior.

   b. Increase range of motion? Yes, that is a specific behavior. It happens also to be the best way to diminish pain in the future.

6. A young woman, diagnosed as "anorexia nervosa" comes with no pattern of vomiting but a consistent pattern of 800 to 1,000 calories a day of dietary intake and a body weight of 72 lbs. What is the behavior to be changed?

   a. Weight? No, that is not a behavior.

   b. Calories taken? No, calories are not behaviors.

   c. Eating? Yes, that is a behavior. (It might be counted as mouthfuls, for example, a point to be considered in the next chapter.)

   In this example, in the interests of brevity, we have not considered why she does not eat more, i.e., the reinforcement for being "skinny," the punishment for being "non-skinny," or the failure of eating behavior to be reinforced. Those issues would need to be clarified and dealt with as well. The point for the moment is that that aspect of the problem having to do with changing eating behavior should focus on eating, not weight or calories.

SUMMARY

The major point of this chapter is the importance of being precise about what behavior is to be changed. Vague and general statements do not define targets. We must be precise and pinpoint the behavior that is to be increased and decreased.

4
MEASURING BEHAVIOR—THE MOVEMENT CYCLE

STATEMENT OF THE PROBLEM— UNITS OF BEHAVIOR

In order to change behavior, you need to know both what the behavior is and how often it occurs. In the preceding chapter we made the point that you need to be precise about what behavior you are going to change. To be precise you must have some unit of measurement by which to state how much or little of the behavior that you want to change is presently occurring. A convenient unit of measurement or description of behavior is the movement cycle.

MOVEMENT CYCLE—DEFINITION AND EXAMPLES

A movement cycle is simply one full sequence of the behavior. A movement cycle ends when the person is in a position to repeat the behavior. For example, in walking, the movement cycle is left foot *and* right foot. If you counted just the left foot movement, the person would not be able to repeat until he or she had also moved the right foot. Consider smoking. The movement cycle in smoking could be the puff; that is, the smoker, after having inhaled *and exhaled,* is in a position to repeat the behavior.

COMBINING MOVEMENT CYCLES

Movement cycles can be combined into larger units if it is convenient to do so and if in doing so your behavioral analysis does not become too vague. In walking, the movement cycle can be the left-right unit. Suppose you are dealing with a patient who is just beginning to take the first few hesitant steps. In that case, the left-right unit is probably the best movement cycle. Each pair of steps can be counted. You might ask, why not count each single step; that is, each time the left foot comes forward is one, and each time the right foot comes forward is another. The problem, however, is that your patient may venture the left foot forward, hesitate, return it, and then repeat. Has walking occurred? No. But when the left and then the right foot are brought forward, and the person is in a position to take another step, walking has occurred.

A behavior change program with a patient might include increasing walking. After the first few days, he or she builds up from a step or two to perhaps 50 or so steps before rest is needed. At that point you might change the movement cycle or unit of measurement of walking. You could combine steps into distance measures by marking with colored tape two points, which are 25 feet apart, on the ward corridor. Your patient could begin to walk laps between these two points. The movement cycle then becomes a lap, which in this case equals the round trip of 50 feet. Remember, you want the round trip so that the patient is in a position to repeat. Later on, as the patient progresses (and gets tired of walking the same course all of the time), you can combine movement cycles into still larger units. Once around the ward may be 200 feet, and that can become a lap.

Let us consider again the smoker. The smallest movement cycle for smoking would be the puff. It would make sense, however, also to use as a movement cycle the number of cigarettes smoked. In that case, the movement cycle could become a cigarette lighted, smoked, and extinguished. Ordinarily, you would not need to worry about whether every cigarette was smoked down to the same length. Over a period of time that would average out. If for any reason that was something to be concerned about, you could always go back to the smaller and more precise movement cycle of the puff. Similarly with walking, you could always go back to number of steps instead of number of laps if more precision and detail are needed.

When smaller units of a behavior are combined to form a larger unit or movement cycle, care must be taken to limit the movement cycle to a single kind of behavior. For example, we combined pairs of steps into laps where we were concerned with walking. Our larger unit was concerned solely with walking. We did not, for example, use "morning activities" as our new and larger movement cycle. Morning activities include walking, perhaps; but they also include a lot of other things. More important, if we content ourselves with "morning activities," we could not specify whether any walking had occurred. Our patients might have sat all morning. When we combine smaller units into larger movement cycles, we are combining only units of the behavior to be changed, not other behaviors also.

SUMMARY

1. To change behavior you need to count it.
2. To count it you need a unit of measurement: the movement cycle.
3. A movement cycle occurs when the person has completed a unit of the behavior so that he is in a position to repeat it.
4. Smaller units of behavior can be combined into larger units to make up a movement cycle so long as the movement cycle continues to include only one kind of behavior.

RATE OF BEHAVIOR—DEFINITION AND EXAMPLES

In addition to the movement cycle, there is another important unit of measurement we must use. We need to know both how much of something was done and in how long a *time period*. Perhaps you are concerned with increasing fluid intake in a patient who needs to keep the bladder and kidneys flushed out. Your target fluid intake level would not be 4,000 ml; it would be 4,000 ml *per day*. For the smoker, it is not 35 cigarettes; it is 35 cigarettes *per day*. For the walking patient, it is not 12 200-foot laps, it is 12 200-foot laps in, for example, a 1-hour walking session. In short, we need to know the *rate* of behavior; that is, the number of movement cycles per some unit of time. The unit of time can, of course, vary from situation to situation. In the example of walking laps, it might be the number of laps walked per morning or per hour or per day. Whichever time unit you use, you must stick to it for that patient. You should not measure it as 12 laps per hour one day and 12 laps per day the next.

Some further examples help illustrate these points. Mr. Y was an elderly stroke patient who experienced difficulty feeding himself. After many difficulties and failures, he gave up trying. His nurse sat down with him and worked out a treatment plan to increase self-feeding behavior. She needed a unit of eating behavior that was much more precise than the general statement, "he does not feed himself." She chose as the movement cycle the mouthful, defined as loading a fork or spoon, moving it to the mouth, unloading it, and returning it to the food or the table. It was now possible to specify how much or little self-feeding Mr. Y accomplished. For two meals the nurse counted the number of movement cycles carried out by the patient. That gave the baseline, or starting point, for the efforts at changing his self-feeding behavior, which in this case was zero. The nurse also determined that Mr. Y was capable of feeding himself, even though it was a bit arduous for him. She then worked out a treatment plan with him involving the use of reinforcers made contingent upon the target behavior, self-feeding. She chose perhaps the most natural and available of reinforcers in that situation, the mouthful. Each time he took a mouthful, she would help him with a mouthful. In subsequent meals, she reduced the reinforcement schedule. She expected him to take an increasing number of mouthfuls for each mouthful she delivered. Figure 4 shows what happened. This example illustrates a number of points. Keep it in mind when reading Chapter 5 on reinforcers, because this example illustrates the use of naturally occurring reinforcers and the value of reducing reinforcer schedules.

At this point we emphasize that use of the mouthful as the movement cycle permitted a precise statement of how much or little self-feeding was being performed. Also, the nurse showed the rate of self-feeding by reporting the percentage of self-feeding per meal. An even

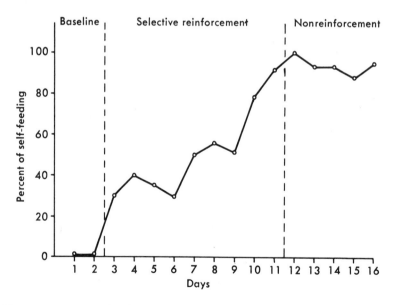

Figure 4. Increased self-feeding in an elderly stroke patient. Reinforcement schedule was gradually reduced as the program progressed.

more precise measurement of rate would have been the actual number of mouthfuls per meal; but in this case that information would add little, because meals vary so much in their size.

Let us consider another example, a 6-year-old, seriously mentally retarded boy, whom we shall call Tim, who was receiving daily physical therapy exercise sessions. Tim screamed almost incessantly for reasons that were never entirely clear, since there was no evidence to indicate that he was in pain. His therapist needed to reduce screaming both because it was obnoxious and disruptive to everyone around Tim and because it interfered with exercising. The movement cycle was the scream, defined as starting *and stopping,* even if stopping was only for a breath. She counted the rate of screaming per minute. Once she knew the baseline—the rate of the behavior at the outset of behavior change program—she tried to change the rate by using her attention as a reinforcer. Each time he screamed, she turned her back on him. It did not work. But she did not make the mistake of assuming that the behavior could not be changed. She recognized that what she hoped would have been an effective reinforcer at that point, her attention, was not. She selected another reinforcer. She equipped herself with a supply of graham crackers, and she ignored his screaming, saying nothing about it. But when he made a sound other than screaming or maintained a few seconds of silence, she reinforced him with a bite of a graham cracker. This quickly produced increased silence and permitted her to shift to where she would reinforce with

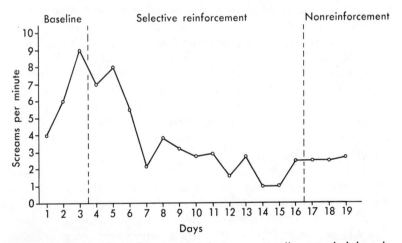

Figure 5. Reduced random screaming in a mentally retarded boy by reinforcement.

graham crackers when specified intervals of silence (or nonscreaming) occurred; for example, 15 seconds, then 30 seconds, then 1 minute. That is, at first a second of silence was reinforced. After some success with that, she required 5 seconds of silence, and so on until Tim would scream only in occasional bursts. His rate during his treatment hours went down to about 2 per minute from the baseline average of 6.3 per minute. These results are shown in Figure 5. His therapist had to discontinue the project before completion because of a change in her work assignment. As a result, when she withdrew the reinforcers on day 18, the rate of screaming went back up part of the way, and she did not have the opportunity to reapply the reinforcement program for a longer interval to more firmly establish the new behavior.

RECORDING FORMS

Use of these methods should not become so cumbersome as to negate or outweigh the performance advantages they offer. On the other hand, effectiveness of the methods requires precision of observation, both in relation to the behavior dealt with and the reinforcers serving as the instruments of change.

Recording behavior and its change serves two functions. (1) It permits the professional to identify present behavior in order to determine what to change, whether or not the behavior is changing, and whether or not the program needs modification. (2) Recording can itself become a form of reinforcement. The patient, family members and visitors, and professional staff may all realize encouragement or reinforcement from observing a visible record of behavior and behavior change. This second function, the display of results, will be considered in Chapter 5.

Figure 6 illustrates a form on which have been recorded a number of treatment or exercise activities each day by a patient being treated for chronic pain. The columns show each set of behaviors to be recorded and the rows for each time interval or treatment session: hour, day, or week, as indicated. This kind of form is useful when reinforcement is not being recorded.

Forms such as these may be carried by patients as they move from one treatment station to another, if they are in a setting, in which several behaviors are under systematic change. The patient should be given a firm-covered folder in which to carry the forms. The very presence of the folder, in fact, helps to remind both patient and therapist to keep good records.

As long as the patient is mentally and physically competent to

Prescribed exercises

Date	AM/PM	Laps (200)	Bicycle .1	Let-backs	Pelvic tilt	Knee to chest R	Knee to chest L	Hip abduction R	Hip abduction L	Hip extension R	Hip extension L	O.T. Loom (rows)	O.T. Turkish knot rug
	AM	8/8	1.5/1.5	6/6	12/12	10/10	10/10	6/6 5#	9/9 8#	8/8 7.5	10/10 10	16	12
	PM	8/8	1.5/1.5	6/6	13/13	10/10	10/10	7/7	10/10	9/9	5/5 12.5	16	12
	AM	9/9	1.6/1.6	7/7	14/14	11/11	11/11	8/8	5/5 10#	10/10	6/6	17	13
	PM	9/9	1.6/1.6	7/7	15/15	11/11	11/11	9/9	6/6	5/5 10	7/7	17	13
	AM	10/10	1.7/1.7	8/8	16/16	12/12	12/12	10/10	7/7	6/6	8/8	18	14
	PM	10/10	1.7/1.7	8/8	17/17	12/12	12/12	5/5 8#	8/8	7/7	9/9	18	14
	AM	11/11	1.8/1.8	9/9	18/18	13/13	13/13	6/6	9/9	8/8	10/10	19	15
	PM	11/11	1.8/1.8	9/9	19/19	13/13	13/13	7/7	10/10	9/9	5/5 15	19	15
	AM	12/12	1.9/1.9	10/10	20/20	14/14	14/14	8/8	5/5 12.5#	10/10	6/6	20	16
	PM	12/12	1.9/1.9	10/10	20/20	14/14	14/14	9/9	6/6	5/5 12.5	7/7	20	16
First quota		8	1.5	6	12	10	10	6	9	8	10	16	12
Increment		1/Day	.1/Day	1/Day	2/Day	1/Day	1/Day						
Goal		30	3.0	20	20	20	20	20/20#	20/20#	20/20#	20/20#	20/20#	16

Patient _____
O.T. _____
P.T. _____

Figure 6. Recording exercise quotas and performance. (From Fordyce, W. E.: Behavioral methods for chronic pain and illness, St. Louis, 1976, The C. V. Mosby Co.)

do the actual recording, it is usually better after the first few days of the program to let the patient take over this task. By then the therapist or nurse should know the patient well enough to be able to judge whether there is likely to be a problem of false recording or cheating. Periodic checking by the professional is usually sufficient to avoid a cheating problem, and patient involvement in treatment is likely to be enhanced by assumption of the recording task.

Some behavior change processes require making explicit the timing and/or number of reinforcements delivered. How to record when using a point or token system is illustrated in Chapter 6.

PRACTICE PROBLEMS
Movement cycles

Try the following examples to practice identifying movement cycles.

1. You want your patient to begin a self-monitored medication regimen. What is the movement cycle?
   a. Taking medications? No, that is too vague, and you cannot identify whether he has completed the task.
   b. Swallowing a pill? Yes, he is in a position to take the next one.
2. An elderly patient needs to be encouraged to practice bed-to-standing transfers. What is the movement cycle?
   a. Increased mobility? No, that is too vague, and you cannot tell when he was in a position to repeat.
   b. Getting out of bed? No, he is not in a position to repeat a bed-to-standing transfer.
   c. Bed-to-standing, then standing-to-bed? Yes, now he can repeat the transfer.
3. A nursing home patient is capable of propelling her wheelchair but waits for someone to push her. What is the movement cycle?
   a. Wheeling herself down the hall? No, that is too vague at the outset.
   b. Pushing forward on the wheelchair wheels, releasing her hands, and returning them to the starting point? Yes, that is a specific unit of the behavior, and she is in a position to repeat it.
4. A patient calls his nurse incessantly. What is the movement cycle?
   a. Thirty minutes of calling without interruption? No, that is too vague.
   b. Number of calls? Yes, you can count them, and he is in a position to repeat after each call.

Rate of behavior

Try each of the following examples to practice identifying rate of behavior.

1. The patient who is beginning a self-monitored medication program has a movement cycle of swallowing a pill. How do you measure his rate of behavior?
   a. Time interval between when medications are delivered and when they are taken? No, that is not the target.
   b. Number of prescribed pills he takes each day or, if more precision is needed, each 4 hours, and so on? Yes, that is the rate you are interested in.

2. The elderly patient who is practicing bed-to-standing transfers has a movement cycle of bed-to-standing-to-bed. What is the rate?
   a. Number of seconds it takes to transfer? No, you are trying to increase the number of times he does it, not how rapidly he does it.
   b. Number of transfers per day? Yes, that is what you are trying to increase. (If more precision is needed, you could use initially as rate the number of transfers he does per 1-hour training session.)

3. You have defined the movement cycle for wheelchair propelling as a push, release, and return of the patient's hands to position for another push. What is the rate?
   a. How fast the wheelchair moves; that is, how many minutes it takes her to go the length of the corridor? No, that is not what you need to measure.
   b. Number of times she propels herself, not how hard she pushes and therefore how fast she goes? Yes, you need to measure how many times she propels herself. As she progresses to increasing numbers of propelling, you can expand the movement cycle to, for example, the number of times she goes the length of the corridor each hour or day.

4. How are you going to measure the rate of the calls of the patient who calls his nurse incessantly?
   a. Cumulative number of calls? No, that is too gross for your purposes.
   b. Number of calls per hour or per nursing shift? Yes, that would give you a quite precise measure.

In this chapter we have emphasized the importance of counting behavior in order to be able to be precise in setting up behavior change programs.

SUMMARY

1. To change behavior you must be able to count it.
2. To count behavior you need a unit of measurement: the movement cycle. A movement cycle occurs when the person has completed the behavior and is in a position to repeat it.
3. Movement cycles may be combined into larger units so long as those larger units continue to focus only on the behavior of interest.
4. In counting behavior there must be both a movement cycle and the rate at which it occurs. Rate is the number of movement cycles per some unit of time.

5
REINFORCERS

As a health care professional, you have a responsibility to identify patient problems and to formulate plans for patient care; you also supervise and help with the performance of the tasks involved. Tools for the management of physical care must be understood, safe, and under control. Similarly, reinforcers, tools for the management of behavioral care, must also be understood, safe, and under control.

DEFINITION

The test question for determining whether something is a reinforcer is, "Does it in fact influence the rate of the behavior it follows?" When a true reinforcer follows immediately after a behavior, the strength or rate of that behavior tends to increase. When a true reinforcer is withdrawn so that it no longer follows a particular behavior, the rate or strength of the behavior tends to decrease. If neither of those occurs, what you thought were key reinforcers for that patient at that time in fact were not. When the behavior continues at the same rate, you can assume reinforcers other than the one you withdrew are the keys to maintaining the behavior.

Because that is so, you cannot automatically assume that something will or will not be a reinforcer. You must try it out; that is, arrange things so that what you expect will be an effective reinforcer will occur only when the behavior you are trying to increase occurs. What is the result? Does the rate of the target behavior increase? If it does, you were correct. What you thought would be an effective reinforcer was just that. If, however, the rate of the target behavior does not increase, you can assume that what you thought was an effective reinforcer in fact was not. In the first chapter we discussed the case of Mary. Her nurses had decided that their attention in the form of chatting with her was likely to be an effective reinforcer by which to help Mary increase use of the commode rather than the bedpan. They made chatting contingent upon use of the commode. Their efforts were rewarded by Mary's increased use of the commode. Their attention was a positive reinforcer for Mary. Had Mary continued to call for the bedpan as often as before, her nurses would have had to conclude that their attention was not enough of a positive reinforcer to serve as an effective tool in helping Mary to change her behavior toward more independent living and that some other reinforcement was continuing to maintain bedpan behavior.

If something is a positive reinforcer, the behavior upon which it was contingent will decline in rate if that reinforcer is withdrawn. That was illustrated in the example of young Bert, who messed his pants. His parents withdrew attention as a contingency to "messing behavior" and were responsive when Bert used the bathroom. The expectation that parental attention would influence Bert's behavior proved correct, which of course does not surprise us.

Remember that a positive reinforcer is something that in fact increases the rate of a behavior when it is made contingent upon occurrence of that behavior. Similarly, a positive reinforcer is something that in fact decreases a behavior if the reinforcer is withdrawn so that, although it used to follow when the behavior occurred, it now no longer does so.

CONTROL

If you cannot control a reinforcer, do not use it. Control of a reinforcer means that the reinforcer occurs only when the behavior to be increased has occurred. Suppose, for example, you have an elderly patient who lives in a nursing home and who likes to play checkers. Suppose also that he needs the exercise of walking to the dayroom and he has instead begun spending nearly all of his time in bed. If visitors, family members, volunteers, or nursing staff come to his bedside to play checkers with him while he remains in bed, playing checkers cannot be used as a reinforcer for walking behavior. He receives the reinforcer (checkers) whether he walks or not; that is, a game of checkers is not contingent upon walking. If, however, a plan is worked out whereby everyone agrees that Mr. X will be offered a checker game *only* when he walks to the dayroom and that he will in fact receive such an offer if he walks to the dayroom, checkers can be tried as a reinforcer designed to help increase walking. Under those conditions a game of checkers can be made contingent upon occurrence of the behavior it is designed to influence, walking; in other words, delivery of a checker game can be controlled.

In Chapter 2 we described how Mr. B had decided to use a before-dinner cocktail as a reinforcer to increase bladder output at a certain time. Mr. B had his own supply of liquor, but he placed that liquor under control of the behavior change process in which he was engaged. If he achieved his quota of bladder output, he received the reinforcer. If he failed to meet his quota, he would not let himself have a cocktail. Suppose he was worried about his own ability to succeed in this particular behavior change process and therefore decided to give himself a special encouragement to continue to participate by taking a cocktail when he failed to meet his bladder output quota. Had he done that, we have every reason to expect that the behavior change process would have failed. Instead of having improved his chances by encouraging himself, he would have removed the effectiveness of a cocktail as a reinforcer by letting it become noncontingent; that is, by allowing himself the cocktail whether the behavior to be increased occurred or not.

To understand further the importance that the reinforcer be contingent, consider what would happen if paychecks were delivered on the last day of each month whether or not the behavior—work—that those monetary reinforcers were designed to support and increase occurred. However dedicated they may be to their jobs, it appears unlikely that large numbers of people would show up for work each day and put in a full shift if their paychecks came no matter what they did.

If the reinforcer cannot be controlled, do not use it.

There is a second important aspect to the control of reinforcers: their availability. If the reinforcer cannot be made available when the behavior to be increased has occurred, there is no point in using the reinforcer. The behavior change process requires both that the reinforcer *not* occur when the behavior to be changed does not occur and that the reinforcer *does* occur when the target behavior does occur. That in turn means that the choice of reinforcers must take into account the ability of the system to deliver those reinforcers. If attention is to be the reinforcer chosen, unless the nursing staff can deliver attention at the appropriate times, the behavior change program will not work. In the example of Mary and use of the commode, her nurses were determined that they were going to carry through with the project, both to help Mary and to ease their own load by giving Mary more independence. In the early stages of the project, they carefully arranged that someone would go in to chat for a few moments with Mary when she used the commode.

Consider again the example of the nursing home patient for whom checkers in the dayroom was to be used as a reinforcer to try to increase his getting out of bed and walking. If, when he reached the dayroom during the first few trials at such a program, there had been no one present and ready to play checkers, we cannot expect that the behavior change project would have succeeded.

To recapitulate: instead of assuming that something will effectively reinforce a behavior, be ready to use trial and error to find out. When a tentative reinforcer is selected, be sure it can be controlled. Delivery or occurrence of the reinforcer should be only when the behavior occurs; that is, when the reinforcer is contingent upon the behavior it is designed to increase. When trying to reduce the strength of a behavior by withdrawing a reinforcer from it, you must be certain that the reinforcer will not occur following the behavior. In order for a reinforcer to be effective either in increasing or decreasing a behavior, it must be contingent, or controlled.

SPEED

How important is the amount of time that passes between occurrence of the behavior to be reinforced and delivery of the reinforcer? The answer is clear: the sooner the reinforcer occurs following the behavior it is designed to reinforce, the more effective it will be. Immediately is better than 10 seconds; 10 seconds is better than 1 minute; 1 minute is better than 1 hour. In the early stages of a behavior change process, when the new behavior is just beginning to occur, it usually is crucial for the reinforcer to follow the target behavior immediately. Intervals of even a few seconds between behavior and reinforcer well could result in behavior change program failure. In the early stage of Bert's parents' efforts to help him with his toilet-training problem, when he performed appropriately (that is, in the toilet), his parents made every effort to make one of themselves present in order to be attentive and give praise as soon as possible. In Chapter 1 we examined the case of Mrs. L, who needed to drink more fluids. Before the behavior change project was begun, the usual pattern was for attention (even in the form of exhortation) to occur the morning after the small fluid intake of the preceding day. The clipboard she carried with her served to remind the staff to offer her fluids and, most important, to be responsive when she drank fluids. The clipboard she then began to carry throughout the day made it more certain that staff attention and praise would occur immediately following the behavior to be increased: drinking.

Example—speed of reinforcing

Suppose you have a rather severely brain-damaged male patient, perhaps a young man injured in an auto accident or an elderly man in a convalescent center or nursing home. Your patient may engage in much touching-grabbing behavior, something that is not uncommon in severely brain-injured patients. Each time you come within reach, he seeks to grab your arm or leg. Perhaps he makes some crude amorous advance by trying to grab or pinch. Perhaps his grabbing behavior is more that of a very uncertain and confused person who wants to make sure someone is present and ready to help him by grabbing and holding the passerby. His grabbing behavior is at least irritating. If he is persistent at it, he prevents you from carrying out other duties. He may become so obnoxious or irritating that you find yourself avoiding him, or at least giving him a wide berth as you go about your duties. Clearly, his needs are not going to be served if his behavior results in less rather than more human contact and interaction. You need to help him decrease grabbing behavior or increase greeting-without-grabbing behavior. You, of course, first try to help him by asking him to stop such behavior, but we shall suppose that does not work, as is often the case. Next, you sharpen your tone and tell him to stop. We shall assume that that also fails. You then decide to program your attention as a potential reinforcer to see if you can help him change this self-defeating behavior. You tell him what you are going to do. Specifically, you explain the importance of the behavior change, of how, unless his grabbing behavior changes, he is likely to receive less attention and help, not more. You also tell him that when he grabs at you, you are immediately going to walk away. You also explain that if he does not grab at you when you approach you will stay and talk with him a moment and, if he needs help with something, try to give him that help. By such an approach you have begun to program a reinforcer, your attention, which you can pretty well control. Equally important, you keep in mind that the reinforcer must be delivered promptly following the behavior to be increased: greeting-without-grabbing behavior. During the next few days, you make every effort to walk away from him if he grabs for you.* But should you walk past him while on another errand and he sees you but does not grab, you pause for a moment and tell him you are busy right now but will be back in a moment to talk with him. Minutes later

---

*This does not mean that you should walk away from your patient if to do so would immediately endanger his health. If nursing necessity requires your presence with him, and he grabs, by all means carry out your nursing responsibilities. So far as possible, however, do so in a noncommittal, nonsocializing manner.

you return. You are busy and probably can take only a moment, but you do take that moment to exchange a comment or two with him. When duties bring you directly to him and he does not grab, you make a particular effort to chat pleasantly with him while you are carrying out whatever task brought you to him. Instead of this procedure, had your plan been to reinforce his nongrabbing behavior by coming around at the end of each shift to spend some time with him, it is likely that you would have failed. Later on, after some reduction in grabbing behavior has occurred, you can probably begin to "save up" your attention as a reinforcer to deliver it in a cluster at the end of a shift. Methods for doing that are illustrated in the next chapter. At first, however, your patient will need rapid reinforcement. In carrying out this project, you must communicate closely with your colleagues on each shift, explaining specifically how you propose to proceed. Should anyone fail consistently to program attention in the manner described, he or she will continue to be burdened with the grabbing behavior. Even then, you can expect change on your shift.

We all recognize, when we reflect on the matter, that it is important to provide rapid reinforcement to any learner in the early stages of the learning process. The youngster starting the first grade of school is not effectively reinforced if told that good things will happen upon graduation from college 16 years hence if he or she studies hard now. The adult who begins to learn how to play bridge will not enjoy the game if the earliest experiences at the card table are laden with abstract do's and don'ts or admonitions from others at the table about the mistakes being made. If the other card players really are interested in helping the novice get to the point where he or she can and will play bridge, they will make every effort to introduce the complexities of the game a bit at a time, while offering both encouragement and positive response as each hesistant step is taken along the way. The homemaker bride who greets her breadwinner groom at the door at the end of the work day with a string of problems or complaints is not likely thereby to effectively reinforce coming-home-on-time (or coming-home-at-all) behavior. The groom is similarly not likely to effectively reinforce his bride's behaving-like-a-homemaker behavior by failing to provide positive reinforcement for his bride's halting and unskilled efforts at cooking. Moreover, the time to reinforce cooking behavior is when he is eating, not an hour later.

SUMMARY

What then are the essential characteristics of reinforcers? To summarize:

1. Effectiveness. A reinforcer must influence the rate of the behavior it is programmed to influence. If the rate of the target behavior does not change, reinforcers must be changed.
2. Control. A reinforcer must be controlled. The reinforcer occurs contingent upon the behavior that it is programmed to increase; or, when a behavior is to be decreased, the reinforcer does not occur when the behavior to be decreased occurs. The reinforcer must be available. Promises will not suffice.
3. Speed. A reinforcer must be delivered promptly after the behavior it is programmed to increase.

SELECTION OF REINFORCERS

At this point perhaps you are apprehensive about the complexities of reinforcers and their selection. In actual practice, the selection of reinforcers is usually a straightforward process if a few simple rules are kept in mind. We have said that reinforcers must be effective, controlled, and rapid. There is really only one other important principle to keep in mind with regard to the search for reinforcers. Fortunately, that principle makes your task much easier. David Premack some years ago (1959) made the observation that high-strength behavior may be used to reinforce low-strength behavior. That is now known as the Premack Principle. The Premack Principle states that what a person does a lot of (high-strength behavior) is likely to prove an effective reinforcer by which to increase the rate of what he or she does not do very much of (low-strength behavior). For example, if you were concerned about getting a youngster to do chores around the house (low-strength behavior), you might try to arrange things so that something he or she really likes to do and does a lot of, such as watching television (a high-strength behavior), becomes contingent upon doing chores. In other words, TV time can be earned by doing chores. Similarly, the dieter who has trouble staying on a diet (the low-strength behavior of stopping eating before too much is taken in) may set up an incentive system whereby things he or she really wants badly (high-strength behaviors) are earned by staying on the diet. Consider once again the case of Mary and use of the commode. Her nurses had observed that she liked to chat or socialize. Socializing for Mary was a high-strength behavior. Her nurses arranged things so that high-strength behavior, socializing, became available immediately upon occurrence of commode use, the low-strength behavior to be increased.

Consider the Premack Principle in relation to smoking. In view of the health issues involved, it is difficult to imagine a situation in which one would want to use cigarettes as a reinforcer. If you did for any reason decide to try cigarettes as a reinforcer, you would make the attempt only with a cigarette smoker. For a smoker, smoking is a high-strength behavior, and as such, it might be used as a reinforcer to try to increase the rate of some low-strength behavior. If the person you were working with was not a smoker, cigarettes would not be an effective reinforcer.

Examples—use of the Premack Principle

Suppose you had a stubborn, contentious elderly bachelor on your ward. He recently has had hip surgery. It is time for him to begin walking; but he feels weak, and he has pain when he walks. Perhaps he is afraid to walk. When his nurses approach him to help him out of bed so he can take a few steps around his room or down the corridor, he greets them with bitter arguments about how weak he is and how much it hurts when he tries to walk. You have also observed that he tends to be a "loner." He has few visitors and does not seem to mind: He shows little interest in engaging in conversation with you when you bring him medications. He is simply not interested in socializing with others, preferring instead to lie in bed reading and watching TV. The low-strength behavior to be increased is walking. But what about a reinforcer? Neither attention nor praise seems likely to be effective because he makes it clear that socializing or interacting with others is not a high-strength behavior. He much prefers to be alone. Using the Premack Principle, you ask yourself, "What are his high-strength behaviors that might serve as reinforcers?" And, of course, the answer is that he shows you what some of his high-strength behaviors are by doing a lot of reading and TV watching. Since he likes to be alone to do those things, you negotiate with him. Pointing out the importance of gradually increased walking to his own progress, you suggest that an easy way for him to keep nurses from coming in to coax and hound him to walk is to walk. You suggest to him that he can easily earn privacy and uninterrupted reading and TV watching by short walking sessions. With guidance from his doctors as to how much he should walk, you work out a plan whereby initially each walking session of 10 steps (movement cycle—a left-right pair of steps) earns him 2 hours of time alone to read before the next of the four-per day walking sessions begins. As his strength increases, the sessions are expanded to increasing numbers of steps. Perhaps, for example, you plan it with him so that each walking session he adds 2 steps during the first week, 10 steps the second week and so on. You have put the Premack Principle to work to help your patient. You have put his high-strength behaviors, isolated reading and TV watching, to work strengthening a low-strength behavior, walking.

Earlier in this chapter we considered the example of the patient who grabs at passersby. By that very behavior such a patient shows you that attention or proximity or opportunity somehow to interact with others is a high-strength behavior for him. As was illustrated, you can put that observation to work to help reduce the grabbing behavior by letting attention or socializing be programmed as a reinforcer. Even if, in such a patient, the grabbing behavior is clearly "dirty old man" behavior, it is quite likely that attention or socializing in the form of casual conversation will serve as an effective reinforcer. The following example illustrates this point. The patient was in an exercise program in physical therapy. Each time his therapist approach him to assist him with his exercise, she was subjected to any of a variety of "dirty old man" behaviors, both verbal and physical. Repeatedly he had been asked to stop such behavior but with no

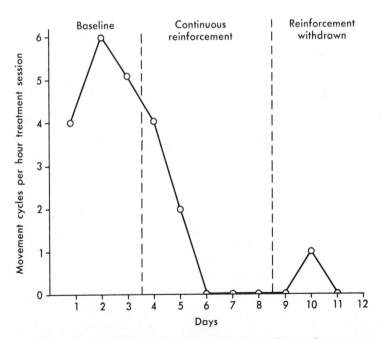

Figure 7. Decreased "dirty old man" behavior by reinforcement.

significant effect. She then decided to make a systematic effort to change this unfortunate and obstructive behavior. She knew by his behavior that he valued her presence and that that was something more than simple "lecherous intent." He valued social interaction. The behavior to be increased (the low-strength behavior) was interacting with her without the "dirty old man" component. The high-strength behavior she programmed as a reinforcer was the broader class of activity: social interaction. Simply stated, the therapist arranged things so that social interaction with her became contingent upon the low-strength behavior occurring—that he stop the obnoxious behavior. Figure 7 shows the results. First, she used three sessions to obtain a baseline. Thereafter, she explained to him that if he engaged in the undesired behavior, she would leave so that his exercises would have to be done in isolation. If, however, he proceeded with therapy tasks without the obnoxious behavior, she would remain at his side while he worked. As shown in Figure 7, the rate of the undesired behavior dropped rapidly. After 5 days, she decided to assess whether his behavior change seemed ready to persist. She decided that for a few days if any of the "dirty old man" behavior recurred, she would no longer withdraw from his presence. On the second day of this test period, following termination of contingent reinforcement by her presence (day 10), there was one minor episode and no more, and the next day it did not recur. She, therefore, terminated her formal recording, satisfied the behavior change had been accomplished.

Suppose you have a patient who argues with you each time you bring her medications. She complains about their taste, about the quality of care in the hospital, about the weather, about breakfast, about her mattress. Bringing her medications becomes an arduous chore. She often refuses to take her medications, and the only way you can get her to cooperate is to cajole her. If you work at it hard enough, you usually succeed; but you often feel as though you have been put through a wringer. How can you get her to quit arguing about taking medications? Sometimes that kind of arguing behavior occurs because it increases the patient's chances that someone will spend time with her: If she does not argue, her nurse will deliver the medications and proceed with her rounds; if she does argue, she keeps her nurse closeby for at least a few minutes. In such instances, the high-strength behavior is interpersonal contact or attention. Using the Premack Principle, you can put that high-strength behavior to work to, in a sense, reduce itself. You might try saying to your patient, "Here are your medications. I'll come back in a few minutes. If you have taken them, we can spend a few minutes talking about some of these problems. I can't spend the time now to argue with you because I have other patients due for their medications, so I'll just leave them here on your bedside stand while I go around the ward." In such an arrangement you are testing whether attention and interpersonal contact are high-strength behaviors by which to reduce arguing. In situations of this sort, it may be that you have reason to believe your patient would throw the medications out the window, hide them and take too many at one time, or pour them down the sink instead of taking them. In that case, instead of leaving the medications on the bedside stand when she refuses to take them, say to your patient, "I'll come back in a few minutes with your medications. If you feel ready then to take them, since I'll have my medication rounds out of the way, I'll be able to spend a few moments with you so we can discuss some of these problems."

The Premack Principle is one of the most useful behavior change tools. A few minutes of reflection about any given patient will almost always reveal some high-strength behaviors he or she displays that might be programmed to help make a behavior change.

NATURAL VERSUS EXOGENOUS REINFORCERS

We usually think of reinforcers as rewards or incentives. However, it is probably true that most people think of many rewards or incentives only as special things, such as money, a new dress, ice cream, a vacation, or a trip to the zoo. These examples of reinforcers are consequences that occur by special arrangement; they do not occur naturally in a situation, but only when special arrangements are made. They can be considered as exogenous, or not a natural part of the situation. In contrast, in many of the examples thus far presented, the reinforcers used were things or events that were a natural part of the situation. For example, nurse attention is a natural part of good nursing care. It occurs in every treatment setting. Similarly, in Chapter 4 the program with Mr. Y was discussed in which his nurse used helping with feeding as a reinforcer to help him increase self-feeding. In that case, help with feeding was a naturally occurring part of the treatment setting. It was what she had been doing before beginning Mr. Y's behavior change project.

Reinforcers can be natural or exogenous. The Premack Principle calls your attention to naturally occurring reinforcers. If someone is doing a lot of something, that behavior is, by definition, a natural part of the setting; it occurs without special arrangement. Clearly, naturally occurring reinforcers are useful things to know about because it means that they are already available and only await programming to make them contingent upon the behavior to be changed. Your job as a behavior change agent is made immeasurably easier by this fact. It is very often the case, in helping a patient change some of his or her behavior, that effective reinforcers are already a natural part of the situation and need only to be identified and programmed to be put to work to help the behavior change process. You often do not need to look about to make some special arrangement, such as a bottle of beer, rental of a TV set, special visitors, or a new magazine in order to find effective reinforcers.

In this chapter examples have been cited in which naturally occurring reinforcers were used to help a patient change behavior. One patient was helped to increase walking and activity level by arranging for a checker game in the dayroom—something that already was available in the situation. Another patient was helped to increase walking by being permitted to read or watch TV in isolation, something that was already occurring in the situation. One patient was helped to reduce grabbing and another to reduce "dirty old man" behavior by selective presence and attention from his nurse or therapist. Presence and attention were naturally occurring events and needed only to be programmed on a contingent basis to help change behavior.

The importance of this point and of the Premack Principle, which supports it, cannot be overstated. The search for reinforcers is usually an easy matter that does not require arduous arrangements or special resources in order to help your patients change behavior. In short, no matter how deprived the situation, one can nearly always find some high-strength behavior that is a natural part of the situation and that, when programmed systematically on a contingent basis, can serve as an effective reinforcer. Moreover, because of the power of the Premack Principle, you, as a behavior change agent, need not feel that behavior modification is difficult to do or is a process requiring elaborate resources and arrangements in order to succeed.

ATTENTION AS A REINFORCER

The principal natural reinforcer we have thus far considered has been attention, programmed in such forms as socializing, chatting, and therapist presence. The appropriate and constructive use of attention is one of the most helpful tools that nursing personnel have by which to help their patients. In most situations attention meets the criteria for a good reinforcer. In settings of chronic illness and disease it is particularly likely to be an effective reinforcer. When attention is contingent upon a particular behavior, the rate of that behavior will probably increase. When attention is systematically withdrawn as a consequence to a particular behavior, the rate of that behavior will probably decrease, as was seen in Figure 6, where therapist attention was withdrawn when "dirty old man" behavior occurred. Attention can usually be controlled when all the nurses work together so that their interacting with the patient makes their attention contingent upon the behavior to be increased. Attention is also available. A short-handed ward crew or nursing home staff often cannot provide nearly as much attention as they would like, but they can nearly always provide some attention, which can therefore be programmed to occur systematically to help a patient. Finally, attention is something that potentially can be delivered very rapidly. A nurse cannot always stop at once to chat with a patient, but can nearly always pause long enough to reassure him or her that she will return at a particular time to chat.

REST OR TIME OUT AS A REINFORCER

In addition to attention, there is another naturally occurring reinforcer in almost every health care setting (including homebound self-care programs) that often can be programmed to help the behavior change process: that is rest, or time out. When an activity is unpleasant or fatiguing or painful, we periodically give ourselves a rest. We take a few moments of time out from the activity. The hiker on a mountain trail pauses every once in awhile to sit on a log beside the trail to catch his breath. The secretary takes a coffee break. The busy nurse pauses for a moment in the nurse's station. The grade school student gets time out in a recess period in which to go outside to play with classmates. In each case, a period of activity that may (or may not) be arduous, difficult, unpleasant, or fatiguing is followed systematically by rest or time out. Using the Premack Principle as a guide, we can see that the hiker, the secretary, the nurse, and the student showed by their actions that intervals of rest and time out were high-strength behaviors. In each case, rest and time out were naturally occurring events that were available, potentially subject to control, and capable of being delivered promptly following work or effort. Under those conditions, rest and time out clearly meet the criteria for being potentially effective reinforcers. In health care settings, as in nearly any other kind of setting in which behavior change efforts are under way, rest or time out is potentially available as a convenient and naturally occurring reinforcer by which to help people change behavior. Perhaps even more frequently than in the case of the systematic use of attention, rest and time out await only our ingenuity at using them to serve as most helpful aids in the behavior change process.

Example—rest and time out as reinforcers

The case of Freddie, who in his early teens developed multiple brain cysts requiring repeated brain surgery, illustrates the programmed use of rest and time out. He had been a sickly child throughout much of his life. He had been characterized as dependent, passive, and lethargic. Following his most recent brain surgery, his lethargy was even more pronounced to the point where he was described as unmotivated to do anything, which of course was an exaggeration but conveys some idea of how he acted. The problem with which we concern ourselves here was how the treatment team was to get this lethargic young man to exercise in order to strengthen muscle function and increase stamina and coordination. Among other activities that his doctor prescribed were two we shall consider here, pulling wall weights with his arms and riding a fixed bicycle. The early efforts by his therapist to get him to work at those (and other) activities were met by his protest that he was too weak and too tired. Freddie also voiced many complaints about being in a hospital and repeatedly asked his parents and his doctor to let him go home. The Premack Principle was put to work. Freddie made it clear by his behavior that rest and time out from effort and treatment were high-strength, or high-value, behaviors for him at that time. After complete discussion with his parents, the treatment team set up a simple behavior change process by which to use rest and time out, high-strength be-

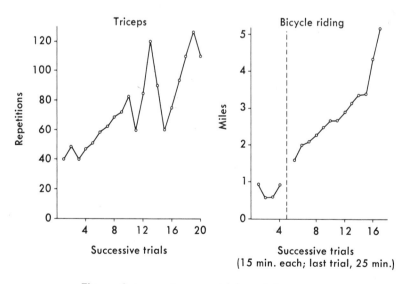

Figure 8. Increasing exercise by reinforcement.

haviors for Freddie, to reinforce pulling wall weights and riding the bicycle, currently low-strength behaviors. A point system was devised. Freddie was given a poker chip each time he met an exercise quota. He could use poker chips to "purchase" either rest from the treatment session or time out of the hospital in the form of weekend passes. An initial baseline was established in the wall weight exercise and bicycle riding from which his therapist by observation knew about how much of each activity he could and would do before stopping from real or feigned fatigue. She then set quotas with him. Initially those quotas were at the baseline level he had already demonstrated. She then awarded him a point (in the form of a poker chip) for meeting the quota. By that method, rest or time out from the wall weight session became contingent upon reaching his quota. She next began adding to the quota by permitting him to earn extra chips for each increment in performance. The more chips he earned the sooner the session ended and the more weekend pass time he could have. Figure 8 shows the results. The graph for the wall weight exercise shows momentary drops in number of repetitions as extra pounds of weight were added to the task, but overall performance rose rapidly.

Example—rest as a reinforcer

Suppose you have a patient with back pain who needs to walk to build up her strength but who finds walking painful if she goes more than a short distance. Let us suppose that her initial walking tolerance is 600 feet. She needs to walk to increase strength, avoid joint con-tractures, and maintain general body tone. Her doctor prescribes walking. It is your job to help her to increase the amount she can and does walk. Using the Premack Principle, you note the obvious: bed rest and time out from walking are very high-strength behaviors for your patient. You encourage her to walk back and forth on a measured 50-foot course marked off in the ward corridor. Since she can walk some distance, you let the movement cycle become 100-foot laps (one round trip on the measured course). As noted, her initial tolerance is 600 feet. By observation you note that when she is asked to "walk to tolerance" she walks approximately six laps. That is her base line. Next, using the Premack Principle, you work out a plan whereby rest or time out from walking, obviously high-strength be-haviors for her since she so much prefers to remain in bed to walking, can become contingent upon the low-strength behavior, walking. To do this you simply plan with your patient that she can return to her bed to rest when she has completed a walking quota. You explain to her that you are well aware of how difficult initially it is to walk more than a short distance. You suggest to her, therefore, that she first practice only small amounts of walking, such as only five laps instead of her initial tolerance level of six laps, before returning to her bed to rest. That arrangement makes rest and time out from walking contingent upon the behavior you are trying to increase: walking. If, instead, you asked her each time to walk to tolerance, quitting only when her pain began or became so severe that she could not continue, you would be delivering the reinforcers of rest and time out contingent upon the behaviors you are trying to decrease: pain or fatigue. You observe your patient as she walks her five laps to meet the initial quotas. After a few trials—for example, in a morning and an afternoon walking session for 3 days—you note that she is walking fairly easily. Praising her for her progress, you now point out to her she is ready to do more because she is getting stronger; so you raise the quota to six laps. Again, rest and time out are contingent upon occurrence of the target behavior: six laps. You continue in this fashion, increasing walking quotas as your patient shows you she is gaining strength. It is nearly always the case in that approach that patients will readily move past their initial tolerance limits. You will have programmed a readily available, naturally occurring high-strength behavior, rest or time out, to help your patient progress. By preparing a simple graph on a sheet of paper taped to the wall beside her bed on which to display the increasing distances she walks, you could add an additional reinforcer, signs of progress and staff praise for it. Whether or not that is done, you have a right to expect that walking tolerance will increase.

Programming rest or time out from an activity that a patient is reluctant to engage in because of pain, fear, fatigue, lack of interest, or whatever will likely prove to be a most useful tool by which to help patients. Not doing the activity is a high-strength behavior at the outset when the patient is tired, fearful, or reluctant. By simple programming this reluctance can be put to work to help. The patient earns what he or she wants to do, rest or time out, by accomplishing increasing amounts of what he or she is reluctant to do, the exercise or activity.

SCHEDULES—DEFINITIONS AND EXAMPLES

At the beginning of this chapter we said that a reinforcer must be under control to be considered an effective tool for behavioral change. An important facet of controlling reinforcers is the *schedule of reinforcement,* which is the prescription as to when a reinforcer should be offered as a consequence of the target behavior. Reinforcement may be presented immediately following the behavior (*continuous schedule*) or after several occurrences of the behavior (*intermittent schedule*). For example, your patient Mr. C may receive your praise each time he completes a left-foot–right-foot movement cycle of walking behavior when he starts to learn to walk again. He is on a continuous reinforcement schedule. Perhaps you continue this schedule until he can perform 10 movement cycles. As he improves, you may decide to praise him only after he has completed 50 movement cycles. Now you have him on an intermittent reinforcement schedule. You have prescribed when he is to receive his reinforcer. First you had your patient on a rich reinforcement schedule, and later you made the schedule leaner until he performed 50 movement cycles before he was rewarded with your praise. Your are enforcing a cardinal rule of reinforcement therapy that sets a goal of spacing programmed reinforcers because to do so makes it more likely that a natural reinforcer will take over. In this case the reinforcement schedule helps Mr. C to progress from 1 step to 50 steps and then to 200 steps. This procedure brings him to the dayroom and the TV. He no longer needs your praise to walk, because he walks to see the TV, which is a natural reinforcer for this TV fan. Without spacing out the reinforcers, saying "good, good" 200 times for 200 steps would wear you out; your patient quickly would get fed up with the term; and he might never have made it to the TV room. As it turned out, you had to reinforce him only a rapidly decreasing number of times, using an intermittent reinforcement schedule.

In the sample case of Mary (Chapter 1), who increased her use of the commode, we find that she was reinforced every time she performed the action, commode use. This is a continuous schedule of reinforcement for her behavior. After Mary had learned to use the commode in the hospital, she was discharged. Her visiting nurse had met with the health care team in the hospital and had agreed to reinforce Mary's independent use of the commode whenever she visited her. This is another example of an intermittent reinforcement schedule.

A *variable ratio schedule* includes a plan of reinforcement after so many responses, but the required number varies about some mean or average. If the mean were 12, the required number of responses for each reinforcer might be scheduled as: 9, 21, 3, 12, 18, 15, 6 (Reese, 1966). It is helpful to be able to organize such a schedule because it may conserve reinforcers that are difficult to give very often. In addition, the schedule might prevent the patient's sloughing off the target behavior immediately after the reinforcer is given since he or she might think that there is no hurry: "I'll get my reward no matter how often I complete the task." The patient who cannot predict when the reinforcer is coming may keep busy more of the time so as not to miss one of the reinforcers.

Interval schedules are based on the passage of time and are also divided into two groups, fixed and variable. For example, Gordy, a 6-year-old patient on the orthopedic ward, has a hard time remembering to stay in proper position so his traction therapy will do him some good. His nurse gives him a big red star for his chart on the wall if he is in good body alignment at each meal time. Gordy gets his stars, but after each meal time he forgets to stay in position until it gets close to the next meal. The nurses change the reinforcement schedule from fixed interval to variable interval. His nurses do his "star check" at different times every 8-hour shift. They know that if they vary the hour of the shift when they do the star check, Gordy will have to remain in good position so as not to miss the unpredictable reinforcer, the red star of honor. It is useful to remember that *extinction* or reduction of a behavior is more difficult if it has been reinforced on an interval schedule.

Another point to remember about schedules is that the amount of the reinforcer is important. The phenomenon of *satiation* predicts that the greater the amount of reinforcement recently received yields an increasing ineffectiveness of that reinforcer. For example, if watching TV is the reinforcer for getting-ready-for-bed behavior, it is not wise to fill or satiate the after-dinner hours with TV. *Deprivation,* or the withholding of a reinforcer, will tend to strengthen it. For example, if your young patient likes hamburgers and gets one for so many exercises completed, it would be prudent to have an agreement that no hamburgers would be served on the regular menus.

There are many forms of reinforcement schedules, and all have a common factor that the schedule must be identified and planned, or it cannot be modified judiciously should the need occur.

SUMMARY

Reinforcers must be:
1. Effective. Something is a reinforcer only if it works; that is, if the behavior it follows increases, or, when withdrawn, if the behavior it did follow subsequently decreases.
2. Controlled. If the supply of a reinforcer cannot be controlled to be delivered only when it is supposed to be delivered, it should not be used as a programmed reinforcer. The reinforcer must be available to be delivered at the appropriate time.

3. Rapid. In order to be effective for initial learning, a reinforcer must also be capable of being delivered immediately following the behavior it is designed to influence.*
4. Scheduled. Additional reinforcer delivery rates can be developed as learning progresses; but whether the schedule is continuous or intermittent, it must be planned.

PRACTICE PROBLEM

A hospitalized patient is being helped to increase exercise, for example, walking an increasing number of laps each morning. Because she is lonely and likes her weekend visitors, one plan that is considered is to make visiting opportunities contingent upon meeting increasing walking quotas. What are the problems with that approach?

a. Is the "visitor" reinforcer likely to be effective? Yes, she has been observed to enjoy visits.
b. Are you able to control that reinforcer? Possibly not, in two different ways. First, family members may (understandably) insist on visiting even if quotas have not been met. Under those conditions, the reinforcer would not be contingent. Secondly, what would you do if visiting time was earned by meeting quotas but no visitors showed up? You would need to be sure visitors would appear if they were "earned."

    The remedy to this problem of making the reinforcer contingent and available would likely require that you meet with patient and family together prior to beginning the behavior change program to elicit their cooperation and agreement to participate in a systematic way. They might, for example, call ahead to determine if visiting time had been earned and, if yes, to be sure to come.

c. The delay between meeting walking quotas on each weekday morning and weekend visitors would almost certainly result in a loss of effectiveness of the reinforcer unless special steps for using delayed reinforcement were put into effect, as illustrated.

---

*In Chapter 6 methods for permitting delayed reinforcement are explained and illustrated.

6

TOKEN OR POINT SYSTEMS
FOR DELAYED REINFORCEMENT

CONTRIBUTIONS OF TOKEN SYSTEMS

Many times it is inconvenient or impossible to deliver a reinforcer immediately following occurrence of the behavior you are trying to help your patient increase. Either the reinforcer cannot be delivered immediately, or if it were, it would so disrupt the patient care process that it would not be practical. For example, in Chapter 3 the case of Lori, the young brain-damaged girl with memory problems, was described. Lori's nurse wanted to help train her to do a variety of self-care procedures, or activities of daily living. Lori had been observed to enjoy listening to her radio in her room in the evenings. Her nurse placed a chart on the wall that listed each ADL task to be performed and that provided spaces in which daily performance of each task could be marked. Each mark earned 10 minutes of radio time, to be collected in the evening. Had the program been set up to provide the 10 minutes of radio time immediately following completion of each task, it would have taken hours for Lori to finish her ADLs. Listening to the radio was an effective reinforcer, and it could be controlled; but to deliver it immediately would have been disruptive to Lori's daily routine. By marking the performance of each task on a chart in Lori's room, Lori's nurse provided a token, or symbol, of the reinforcer. The token served to bridge the time gap between occurrence of the target behavior and delivery of the reinforcer. Had she said to Lori that performance of each task would earn 10 minutes of radio time but had not provided some symbol of reinforcement immediately following completion of each task, she would have failed to follow the cardinal rule of rapid delivery of reinforcement. Given Lori's memory problems, one can of course expect that the interval between morning performance and evening reinforcement would have been too long and therefore fatal to the program. Most people in the early stages of learning or behavior change, not just those with brain damage and memory deficits, would not do as well with delayed reinforcement as they would with immediate reinforcement.

In the preceding chapter the case of Freddie was described, in which he earned time out of the hospital on weekends for his performance in exercise programs. Such an arrangement provided as much as a 5-day interval between performance and reinforcement. It would not have been feasible to provide an hour or so of pass time whenever Freddie met an exercise quota. The use of tokens (in the form of poker chips) delivered immediately following performance provided Freddie with tangible, visible evidence that the much sought-after reinforcers were indeed to become available. Those tokens bridged the time gap. They served as immediately delivered symbols of a reinforcement that would be provided later.

In Chapter 3 Mr. J's program was described, in which he earned visiting time with his girlfriend by performing self-care tasks. His girlfriend worked during the days, but she could visit in the evening. Her visits as a reinforcer could be used only if some kind of token or point system bridged the time gap between morning ADL performance and evening visiting hours. By recording on a wall chart as Mr. J performed, his nurse gave him tangible, visible indication of the delayed reinforcer: a visit with his girlfriend.

The use of the token or point systems in the behavior change process adds much flexibility and versatility. Token or point systems contribute in several different ways. As just noted, token systems provide a time bridge between performance of the target behavior and delivery of a reinforcer that cannot be delivered immediately, or if it were delivered, would be disruptive or burdensome to the patient care process. The use of token systems makes it possible to program reinforcers remote in time or place so that they can be delivered symbolically immediately following patient performance.

There is a second important feature to token systems. The use of a token system makes it possible to relate a series of patient behaviors to a single reinforcer. It is often the case that a nurse will be able to identify only one or two apparently effective reinforcers that might be programmed to help the patient, but a number of behaviors may need to be increased. This point was illustrated in each of the three examples just mentioned. Lori and Mr. J needed to increase the rate of strength of a series of self-care tasks. Their behavior change programs, by going to token systems, made it possible to let the reinforcer of radio time in Lori's case and girlfriend visit time in Mr. J's case be programmed or put to work to influence several behaviors. In Freddie's case, poker chips as tokens served to increase two different exercises.

Example—token system in home care program

Suppose your visiting nurse home care program brings you to a retired, elderly stroke patient who presents you with several problems with which you want to help. He is partially paralyzed on the left side, with precarious balance, and is always at high risk when walking unattended. When he arises at night to go to the bathroom, instead of asking his wife for assistance, he lurches to his feet in the dark and gropes his stumbling way to the bathroom. The risk of fall and hip fracture is great. He needs to be helped and should awaken his wife to gain her standby assistance in the trip to the bathroom. That is the first problem. The second problem is that he is careless and forgetful about bathing and dressing. He often fails to brush his teeth, comb his hair, sponge himself clean, and dress. The third problem is that he needs to walk more in order to avoid joint contractures and to help maintain body tone. He uses as his excuse for not walking more (with his four-legged cane and standby assistance from his wife) that he is not dressed and therefore cannot go outside to walk. You are faced with a formidable task. There are diverse problems to be tackled, and your busy schedule makes it impossible to be present to deliver reinforcers when he performs. In such a circumstance the use of a token or point system offers promise of help. You explore with your patient and his wife what incentives or reinforcers might be programmed to help. You point out to both of them the importance of helping him to do the things he needs to do to get along better. You explain to them how they can help each other by planning a simple incentive system. You draw them out on what things he likes to do that might be programmed as reinforcers. Perhaps the concept of incentives seems a bit abstract and unclear to them, and so they are not successful in thinking of possible reinforcers. You might ask how much he likes to watch TV, and they might agree that he spends, if anything, too much time in front of the TV set. It takes just a few minutes more to pin down that the prime TV time for him is the evening, when he generally watches TV steadily from 6:00 to 9:00

PM. You now have identified a potentially effective, controllable, and available reinforcer. Three evening hours easily break down into 12 15-minute units. Keeping that fact in mind, you analyze the problem behaviors into units. Let us suppose it comes out about like this:

1. *Night bathroom visits, wife called:*
   Averages two per night   2 units
   (Wife not called: minus 2 chips)
2. *Dressing and self-care:*
   Brushing teeth twice daily   2 units
   Taking sponge bath once daily   1 unit
   Dressing in street clothes once daily   1 unit
3. *Walking (outside, wife as standby):*
   To the corner and back (1 lap)   1 unit

   Total   7 units

You want him to succeed. You want to be sure that initial efforts receive reinforcement. Therefore, you do not initially expect total performance in order to receive the full schedule of watching TV in the evening. You work out the contract with your patient and his wife so that each unit of performance earns 2 points. You provide them with a handful of poker chips and a clear plastic cup (perhaps placed on the TV set) into which his wife places earned chips and from which she collects chips as he uses them in the evening. He can now earn 14 poker chips per day and trade them in at the rate of one chip per 15 minutes of evening TV watching (or 4 per hour). As a further safeguard against the hazard of your patient's unattended nighttime bathroom visits, you add the provision that if his wife discovers an unattended bathroom trip, she is to remove two chips from his supply, a procedure known as response cost. You write all of this out in a chart much like that shown above. You post the chart where it is easily found (perhaps by the TV set) but keep a copy for yourself as a reminder. You call the next day and periodically thereafter before your next visit to be sure that things are going all right. Suppose he decides to build up a surplus of chips by walking extra laps and then begins to skip some of the other tasks? Anticipating this, you asked his wife to call if that happened—and she calls. You make two simple adjustments in his token economy. First, you raise the price of TV watching to 3 chips per 30 minutes, or 6 per hour (or, if it appears necessary, to 2 chips per 15 minutes, or 8 per hour). This adjustment has the effect of offsetting his surplus of chips. The second adjustment is to attach a premium to total performance. If he goes through the night without a single unattended bathroom visit, he earns a bonus chip (or two or more, as may be necessary). If he does each of his ADLs, he earns one or more bonus chips. In your initial negotiating with him and his wife, you had been careful to point out that the program you were proposing was designed to improve his performance. Therefore, as a natural consequence of improvement, he should expect that he would be able to do more, and you, in turn, would expect him to do more. That is why you periodically adjust the "pay-off rate" to take into account his increased ability. If you explain that ahead of time, you rarely will experience difficulties when those kinds of adjustments are indicated, for those changes show him that he is progressing.

There is a third feature to token systems to be noted. They make a variety of reinforcers available to be programmed either to a single behavior or a series of behaviors. You are on a token economy system in your work. You engage in a variety of behaviors in the course of your job for which you receive a monthly supply of tokens in the form of a paycheck and which you then trade in on a variety of reinforcers, such as food, shelter, clothing, and recreation.

By going to token or point systems with your patients, you will find that just as you can program a single reinforcer to influence a variety of behaviors, you can also program a variety of reinforcers to influence a single behavior or a series of behaviors. In the preceding example of the retired stroke patient, there were several target behaviors and a single reinforcer. It would have been a simple matter, however, to add other reinforcers to the list of things that could be "purchased" with poker chips. Perhaps your community has a home-bound telephone-calling service whereby volunteers call to chat. If that were the case and your patient liked to chat with people, you could arrange on your biweekly visits to his home to determine how many chips he wished to spend on that activity. His wife would collect the chips. You could call the call service to inform them how many calls had been earned to be delivered during the next 2 weeks. Perhaps that same patient very much enjoyed an occasional afternoon in a golden age club. You might place a premium of several chips on such a visit, always making sure that the rate at which he could earn chips has been adjusted so that he does not become significantly deprived.

It is important to note that behavior modification systems are used to change the behavior as the need arises. You might want this patient to limit fluids after supper or to learn to use the urinal at the bedside at night. The same principles will apply to these behaviors.

Example—token system to reduce incessant calling

Imagine that a hospital ward receives a young lady—we shall call her Jane—with a severe head injury from an auto accident. After being in a coma for several weeks, Jane has regained consciousness and begins the gradual process of relearning self-care, ambulation, and so on. She has major memory problems, and she is easily aroused to anger or to emotional upset, all results of her brain injury. Such a patient offers many complex nursing management problems, but we shall focus on just one: incessant nurse calling. Jane seems to fear being alone and so calls her nurse repeatedly. Moreover, when she calls, if there is not a rapid response, her easily triggered emotions spill over into frantic yelling—perhaps cursing or screaming. Even when calls are answered promptly, memory problems are so severe that she seems not to remember moments later that a nurse was just in to check on her. Any nursing unit could not long do its job unless the frequency of calls were reduced. There is a further complication in that her memory problem is going to require extremely rapid delivery of reinforcers if her behavior is to be influenced. It is out of the question for anyone to expect a nursing staff either to ignore her calls or to be able to respond to them rapidly and consistently.

The team sets about the business of analyzing the behavior to be changed and a method of providing programmed and rapid reinforcement. As a first step, recognizing that Jane is often confused, forgetful, and unsure as to the passage of time, her nurses provide her with a clock with a luminous dial. They place it so she can readily see it and therefore has some basis for judging the passage of time. It is sometimes the case with such problems that no further steps need be taken. The clock provides a basis for knowing how long it has been since someone checked on her. We shall assume, however, that the clock was not enough. The next step is to pinpoint the behavior to be changed, in this case the reduction of calling behavior. The movement cycles are defined as a pressing of the call button or each word or phrase of loud calling, or both pressing the button and calling. For example, "Nurse, come help me!" is one cycle. "Nurse! Nurse! Nurse, come help me!" makes three cycles. It is rarely necessary to worry about whether the movement cycle is each word or each sentence or phrase. The important thing is that each person who is counting uses approximately the same standard. The next step is to set up a chart in the nurse's station, marked off by the hours of the day—all shifts. In the line for each of the 24 hours, whenever Jane calls, a tally is marked. Probably 2 or 3 days of baseline counting will suffice, if there is any consistency from day to day in call rate. If there is marked variability from day to day, probably another 2 days or so of counting will prove useful. When the baseline data are tabulated, it is perhaps noted that the call rate varies markedly according to the time of day or night. She rarely calls out during the day and only very occasionally in the hours from about midnight to morning awakening because she usually sleeps soundly. The problem times are from midafternoon, when her daily treatment routines have ended, until a couple of hours after lights out. The team therefore decides to focus on evening-shift calling. The target of their efforts is to reduce to an acceptable level the number of times she calls during those hours.* The baseline data indicate an hourly average call rate of 20.

The nurses explain to Jane that they recognize fully how difficult it is to be sure that someone will be available when needed and how difficult it is to remember how long it has been since someone checked on her. They further explain to her and her family that what is wanted is to help her to feel more safe and secure and at the same time to help her get better at remembering things. Using the Premack Principle, the nurses easily identify at least one reinforcer: attention. The frequency of her calls makes it quite certain that nurse attention is a very important consequence to Jane. Her nurses explain to her that a program is going to be worked out whereby she can earn extra time to visit with them and with volunteers in the hospital. During those visits she will have a chance to talk about whatever she would like. Perhaps it can also be arranged, if she wishes, for her and a nurse or volunteer to work together on a jigsaw puzzle. Two clear plastic cups are placed on the window ledge close to her bed. One is unmarked but the other has a red marker. Her nurses explain that 20 tokens, poker chips, will be placed in the plain cup at the beginning of each hour. Each time she calls, her nurse will answer the call but will also transfer a chip from the plain cup to the red-marked cup. At the beginning of the next hour, if there are still chips in the plain cup when her nurse comes to replenish the supply, she will remain to visit for a few minutes. If the cup is empty, there will be no visiting time. Because it is so important in the early stages of learning or behavior change that reinforcement be delivered promptly, the staff makes a very special effort during the first few hours of the program to be prompt in visiting her on the hour to give her feedback about how she

---

*The goal is of course not to eliminate her calling. That would be both un-ethical and dangerous. The end product of efforts with her should be to bring her call rate down to an average of something less than five per hour—assuming that her general medical status makes that a reasonable and prudent level.

has done and, if she stayed within her quota, to give her 5 minutes of visit time.

Let us consider separately what happens if she fails and if she passes. First, suppose that during the first hour of the program she fails to meet her quota. As is sometimes the case in such situations, the patient may actually markedly increase the rate of calling. Let us suppose Jane does just that and calls 45 times during the first training hour. Each time someone answers her calls, conversation is held to an absolute minimum. Her nurse finds out what, if anything, is needed and provides it. If the call was only to be sure someone was around who would attend to her, her nurse says to her, "That was call number six. If you can keep your calls to less than 20 we will be back at the end of the hour to spend some time with you." If the baseline counting was at all accurate, Jane should quickly return to approximately the baseline level. If, by the end of the first 8-hour shift she has never succeeded in meeting her quota, a too stringent quota was set. The experience data accumulated are added to the original data, and a new quota is set. In view of the early failures in the program, the new quota should be conservative, that is, well within her reach. The new quota might be set, for example, at an amount exceeded by Jane only 25% of the number of hours for which counting has occurred. Or, if you are pessimistic, let the new quota be only slightly below the highest number of calls recorded for any of the baseline hours. Once mastery begins to occur, it is likely that quotas can rapidly be lowered to more modest levels.

What happens if Jane suceeds? Promptly at the end of the first hour, her nurse goes in, gestures to the clock to show an hour has passed, praises her for her performance, noting that she called only 18 times, transfers the 18 tokens from the marked to the plain cup, and stays for a 5-minute visit. At the end of the visit, she reminds Jane, gesturing to the clock, that she will return at such and such a time to spend some time with her if Jane can keep within her quota of 20 calls. If nurse attention is a very potent force, such a patient is quite likely to reduce her calls markedly not because of her memory since her memory problems will make it difficult for her to keep track of how often she has called but rather because the visible supply of tokens continuously displays her performance. The staff is very careful during the first few hours to be prompt about delivering the reinforcers. If for any reason no one is able to stay for 5 minutes, a point is made to make a brief visit to transfer the tokens for the next hour and to tell her that someone will be back in a few minutes—as soon as possible—to visit with her. Suppose she succeeds three or four times in a row; because there were fewer than 20 calls each hour, tokens unexpended by calls would accumulate. Her nurses can then suggest to her that she save up her tokens so that she can have a longer visit; that is, tokens from the plain cup can be spent for visitor time at the rate of 2 minutes per token. She is quite likely to want to do that after the first few hours. It will not be many shifts later that family visits or some time from a volunteer can be programmed. Jane can show her accumulation of tokens to her family as a mark of progress. They, in turn, should by then have been prompted both to collect tokens when they visit and to praise her for her efforts.

After 2 or 3 days of quotas of 20 calls it is time to help move the patient to the next level of performance. The nurses explain to Jane that she can earn extra visiting time by reducing her call rate even further. For example, 15 to 19 calls earn 1 bonus token in the plain cup, 10 to 14 calls earn 2 tokens, 5 to 9 calls earn 3 tokens, and fewer than 5 calls earn 4 tokens.

In the preceding example, notice that prompt reinforcement was given initially. Adding the feature of the token system made it possible, however, to begin to delay reinforcement as well as to program a series of reinforcers: nurse visit, family visit, and volunteer visit. You are limited only by your imagination in thinkng of yet addtional reinforcers that might become available, contingent upon your patient's accumulating further tokens. A walk outside in the sun, a window box flower bed on the window ledge of the dayroom, ice cream, and so on are all likely to be feasible reinforcers that can, by use of a token system, serve to help patients remember and help nursing staff to avoid the rigors of incessant calling.

In the use of token systems, or any other reinforcement program, as progress occurs, increasing amounts of performance are expected for a given amount of reinforcement. Such an arrangement is the standard in almost every learning or skill acquisition process. Notice, for example, that in public education, grades as one kind of reinforcement are given contingent upon increasingly high levels of performance. What earns an A in fourth-grade arithmetic is considerably less than what earns an A in eighth-grade algebra. What earns a nursing instructor's praise is considerably less for the novice than for the advanced student. Changes in expected performance levels are not "cuts in pay." Quite to the contrary, they are signs of progress.

TREATMENT CONTRACTS

One of the most effective ways to make explicit the objectives of treatment and the methods by which they are to be attained is to develop a treatment contract with your patient. Use of contracts relates closely to the use of token systems because the contract sets forth the target behaviors and the contingencies or reinforcement arranged in relation to those behaviors. Reducing these arrangements to contract form has additional advantages. Perhaps most important of all, the very process of sitting down with your patient to develop and negotiate details of the contract ensures that he or she will be an active participant in the process of goal selection and definition. That step has both ethical and performance benefit. The patient (or in instances of mentally incapacitated patients, his or her surrogate) has the right to participate in this fashion. Additionally, the act of doing so almost certainly will increase involvement in the process and identification with the objectives. In behavioral terms, this is another way of saying that you are helping your patient to increase the reinforcing value of both the programmed reinforcers and of the treatment objectives.

A treatment contract sets forth the behaviors or behavior changes contemplated in the treatment process and the contingency arrangements being set up to help bring them about. The contract makes explicit what the patient is expected to do. The contract also sets forth what the therapist is expected to do, including providing for contingent reinforcers.

Developing treatment contracts, of course, requires that the patient (or surrogate, if indicated) be involved. One cannot simply write out a contract and impose it on the patient. To do that would be both unethical and ineffectual. It would be self-defeating to both patient and treatment team.

We can illustrate development and use of a treatment contract by considering the example of a nursing home patient who had been inactive in her previous living arrangement and who, therefore, needs assistance in increasing mobility and taking greater part in self-care activities. We shall further assume that her previous relative inactivity has resulted in sufficient stiffening of joints to make walking and moving about painful. The pain, the ease of fatigue from inactivity, and the now somewhat established pattern of relying on the help of others in the performance of self-care activities all are barriers to increased independence and mobility. Simply stated, she spends her days in a nightgown either in bed or at a bedside chair, expecting others to bring meals to her there while she sits, lost in fantasy, napping, or watching TV.

The range of target behaviors could be extensive but we shall restrict ourselves to considering the following:

Self-care:
1. Dressing
2. Combing hair

Mobility:
3. Walking laps (50 feet each)
4. Dayroom visits (twice daily)

Eating:
5. Walking to dining room for meals

The patient is not likely initially to expect either to strive for or to accomplish these objectives or target behaviors. We shall assume that the sense of participation toward greater mobility and self-care will itself need to be shaped somewhat systematically. To that end, her daughter is brought into the process for a preliminary discussion. The general outlines of the plan are proposed to the daughter and her assistance is requested. Specifically, she is asked to sit in as treatment objectives and methods are explored with the patient. The daughter is also helped to understand how essential her support is in helping her mother to recognize that indeed she can do many things for herself and will feel much better if she does them. The daughter is also helped to understand that it will take systematic effort to bring this about, including systematic forms of encouragement from her, the daughter.

The next step is to sit down with patient and daughter and discuss what the objectives of working with them might be. We shall, of course, assume that each objective considered is within the repertoire of the patient and is not an activity she can never reasonably be expected to attain.

One of the more helpful ways of opening up consideration of the somewhat painful topic of moving from dependence to greater independence is by asking the patient, "If you were to get better, how would you know it?" If responses are in terms of feelings (e.g., "I'd feel better;" "I'd feel more energetic;" "I'd be less depressed;" "I'd have less pain."), those can be accepted, but you should insist that they also be translated into actions, into things people do. For example, if the response is, "I'd have less pain," you might counter with, "OK, but if you had less pain, what would you do? How would you spend your time?" In this fashion, it is usually a straightforward process to help your patient to focus on objectives precise enough to permit systematic treatment.

In the interests of brevity, we shall assume that the kind of discussion just described leads to agreement on the target behaviors listed above. You should have a pretty good idea of a reasonable list of objectives prior to the discussions, but the final list should indeed be generated within the session.

Once the target behaviors have been defined, the next step is to develop the incentive or reinforcer component to the program. Here again, since we all have been functioning within the framework of various incentive systems pretty much throughout our lives, it is usually not difficult to carry out this component. For example, this aspect of the discussion might be something like this: "We know it will be difficult at first for you to get back to moving around and doing more things. You will feel pain, weakness, and fatigue. We want to do all we can to help. We think that you can help yourself more and we can help you, too, if we work out some incentive systems. For example, you really enjoy your daughter's visits and you enjoy watching TV. Why don't we set it up so that you can earn for yourself those very things you enjoy so much. That way you can help yourself, and we can help you get there." You can then go on to explain that each activity or target behavior can be worked on in very small or gradual steps. Emphasize that you will never ask her to do something she cannot do. At first, there will be just small parts of each task to be done by her, and then, as strength and stamina increase, she can gradually build up the amount she does.

The next step is to spell out the increments to each objective. Thus:

Self-care:
1. *Dressing:* Day 1: 1 garment, unassisted; other garments, assisted.
   Day 2: 2 garments, unassisted, etc.
2. *Combing hair:* Day 1: 10 strokes with comb
   Day 2: 20 strokes, etc. to target level.

Mobility:
3. *Walking:* Day 1: Walking 1 50-foot lap accompanied by nurse for standby assistance, in morning and again in the afternoon.
   Day 2: (and thereafter): Increment of 1 50-foot lap each day, standby provided if and as needed.
4. *Dayroom:* When walking laps reaches 200 feet (four laps, the distance from her bed to the dayroom) walking sessions are supplemented by dayroom visits.
   Day 5: Morning dayroom visit, 30 minutes (ad-lib, beyond)

> Day 6: Morning and afternoon dayroom visits
> Day 7: Morning, afternoon, and evening dayroom visits.

Eating:
> 5. *Dining room:* We shall assume 200 feet from bed to dining room.
>> Day 8: Breakfast in dining room (other meals via tray at bedside).
>> Day 9: Breakfast and lunch in dining room.

The final step is to relate those sequences to contingent reinforcement. The most direct and simple way is to treat each task as a separate and equivalent unit. Accomplishment of each earns one point or token. That is, it is completing the quota or task which earns the token; tokens are not given for each unit of each task. Dressing to the quota level earns one token, not one token per garment put on unassisted.

SUMMARY

The major features of token systems are as follows:

1. Token systems make it possible to delay reinforcement to a more convenient time, to use a variety of reinforcers to try to influence a single behavior, and to use one or more reinforcers to influence a variety of behaviors.

2. Because tokens are symbols and not the reinforcers themselves, it is important early in their use in a behavior change project to be sure that they are delivered promptly. It is sometimes necessary to accompany the token at first with an element of a reinforcer for which they can be traded.

3. To establish a schedule, or "rate of pay," you must remember that success breeds success. At first aim for at least an 80% to 90% success rate; that is, of success by the patient. When in doubt, err in the direction of ensuring that he or she will succeed. If there are 10 tasks to be performed (or one task 10 times), performance of 6 to 8 (or even fewer) will earn tokens. If at first no tokens are earned, ease the standards in order to ensure early success.

4. As progress occurs, adjust reinforcement schedules so that increasing amounts of performance are expected for a given amount of reinforcement.

7
SHAPING

DEFINITION

Shaping is the procedure used to develop a behavior that has a rate close to zero or that only happens at random. Shaping is based on reinforcing nearer and nearer approximations of the target behavior.

SHAPING PROCESS

The shaping process has been described many times in connection with the behavior of retarded, deviant, or brain-damaged individuals. Let us assume you are in a different setting; you are the permanent team leader of a nursing team on a busy surgical ward. The 40-year-old woman admitted today will have surgery tomorrow; she will come back from surgery with an ileostomy. You have in your initial data base that the patient is unwilling to care for this stoma after her operation and hopes that her husband will employ an attendant to do this for her. The husband, who has no resources for an attendant, wants his wife to be independent. Since the wife's and husband's goals differ, you decide to attempt to teach the wife ileostomy care as a routine procedure for her information regardless of who might eventually care for the ileostomy. The problem identified is the patient's inability to take care of it herself or to demonstrate the care for an attendant. The possible reinforcers are praises from husband, nurse, and other staff. You construct a flow sheet of a series of steps or approximations to total ileostomy care, and you include a demonstration kit as a practice model onto which the parts of the ileostomy equipment can be applied. You demonstrate the total procedure and then place a "practice" bag on the patient's intact skin and ask her to wear it for 3 hours for the purpose of determining proper placement of the stoma during the operation. All this time you ignore statements of impending failure by the patient. You mark the skin for the proper position 3 hours later and then ask the patient to remove the appliance with adhesive remover. You praise her and check off this step on the flow sheet on the patient's clipboard. The husband sees the flow sheet and praises his wife.

After the operation the patient practices placing equipment parts on the model and is praised after each small step. The flow sheet is checked off when each step is completed. The same process occurs with the patient as her own model as you praise each successful step; you are careful that the step is small enough for her to succeed each time. Patients who feel unable to perform a difficult manual task or are repulsed by stoma care often need this shaping procedure; they usually express pride in themselves after they succeed.

FADING PROCESS

Fading is a technique of going through a desired activity with an individual and gradually decreasing the instructor's participation. The verbal cues used to effect shaping are gradually removed until the behavior occurs without assistance from the instructor. The above example demonstrated the patient's taking over and the instructor's cues being faded out. The natural reinforcer of the husband's verbalized pride in the patient is likely to maintain the behavior.

Implementation examples

You are on duty on a surgical floor, and a problem for one of your patients after his operation is learning complete self-care regarding his diabetic routine. He is 60 years old and will soon be living alone since his daughter will be moving to another state. You learn from the daughter that her father does most of his routine but has continually refused to inject his own insulin. You learn from your patient that he has been a longshoreman all his life and feels that he will never be able to manage the small insulin syringe with his big hands. He tells you that he tried it once, and he had to put the syringe down and ask his daughter to do it for him. You ask him if he would be willing to try once more if you help him through the steps of learning the procedure; he skeptically agrees. You know that if he can perform this procedure, he will be able to cut down on medical costs. He agrees that he would rather spend the money for gas to go fishing than for someone to come in and give him his insulin. You suspect that some of the reasons he has refused past trials of this procedure may have been that he was anxious about possible failure in front of his daughter, that he might not be able to read the measurements on the syringe, or that he might break the small syringe. You know that effective shaping calls for selecting the right responses to reinforce and knowing how long to reinforce each approximation before moving on to the next. You know your patient quite well, and you determine that you will need to progress with the shaping procedure rapidly because he can become impatient very quickly. You have tested your patient's eyesight by asking him to give you his temperature reading; he does this accurately. You tell him you will be in early the next morning to help him learn to give his own injection. You give yourself an hour and a half before he needs to have his insulin. You have arranged with another nurse to answer your lights while you concentrate on this teaching project. You have chosen this early time because it will be less distracting, it will be too early for the daughter's visit, and it is at a realistic time for this procedure. You bring your equipment into your patient's room after he is seated in a comfortable chair and under a good light. The shaping equipment includes a rubber injection practice model, a series of syringes and needles, and an injection bottle of sterile water. The syringes and needles range from very large to the insulin syringe and needle. You start your patient out with the largest syringe and needle. He practices drawing up the water into the syringe, injecting the rubber model, and performing all the tasks associated with insulin injection. With each approximation of using a smaller and smaller syringe, you offer praise and check off the step on a check sheet that you both can see. He moves quickly along the series of syringe sizes: 50, 20, 10, 5 and 2 ml. Simultaneously he decreases the needle sizes. By the time for his actual injection, he is able to manipulate the small syringe and its needle; he completes the real injection task. The next day he performs the procedure while you stand by. He continues to manage his diabetic routine with intermittent reinforcement from the visiting nurse.

A longer and more complex form of shaping is needed to help the next patient you have, a 70-year-old grandfather, paralyzed on the right side following a recent stroke. His problem is that he needs to dress himself in the morning, and he is having difficulty completing this behavior with the use of only his left hand and with almost nonexistent verbal communication. You have demonstrated the procedure of positioning and putting on the shirt; you have made him a set of drawings of each step in the dressing procedure; he knows you as someone he can trust. Now you are ready to attempt shaping putting-on-the-shirt behavior. You have already shaped his behavior to the point where he can consistently position the open shirt correctly on his lap so he can start to pull his paralyzed hand through the color-coded right sleeve. At this time when he has his right hand through the right sleeve, you reinforce his successful approximation with a "good, good" and a pat on his hand. You give him a gold star for that square of his progress chart, since you know that gold stars were reinforcers for him when he learned self-bathing. He seems to like to show his wife his progress chart when she visits. You do not ask him to struggle putting his shirt on all the way; you help him go through the steps of finishing putting on his shirt and tell him, "Nice practice." You plan three shaping sessions a day: morning, after midmorning rest, and after midafternoon rest. You are careful to move from one step to another as rapidly as possible, because you do not want satiation to occur or the possibility that any approximation might become so firmly established that there is little likelihood for another response to occur. Perhaps the next step will be pushing his sleeve over his elbow, and the next step might be pushing the sleeve up over his shoulder. However, you do not want to progress too rapidly, because you might be demanding a response that is unlikely to occur yet. The patient must experience success with each task, or the behavior will not be reinforced, and it will begin to extinguish. As you help him rehearse all the steps toward the terminal behavior, he is also reinforced by seeing the usefulness of the steps; he had a part in putting on his shirt, not just pushing his sleeve up. This rehearsal gives the patient opportunity to shape his skill before he is asked to do the task independently. The process of shaping steps and practicing the whole process has an advantage over praising the patient for a valiant trial of putting on his shirt without the shaping of the series of approximations. Most patients know when they have succeeded alone and when they have practiced with help; when these two categories are reinforced honestly and separately, the patient becomes trusting of those who work with him. Fradulent or meaningless praise is a serious deterrent to successful behavior modification. This goes along with the mocking behavior of long-term patients who scoff at health care professionals who say, "Hello, how are you?" and rush on by. Many of these patients prefer to ignore professionals who expect a friendly response to an automatic inquiry. We have noted that an orderly who is interested daily in the patient's behalf may be a far more potent reinforcer than a professional consultant who visits once a week. The ideal is when the whole team knows the patient well and supports any behavior modification project going on. This support usually occurs when the team, including the patient, has had a part in the planning of the project.

Such a team project was employed in a rehabilitation center where the patient was asking the team to help him in shaping water-drinking behavior. He was a quadriplegic patient and was concerned about putting on so much weight that he would have increased difficulty with his sliding board transfer from bed to wheelchair and his transfer from wheelchair to car. The team agreed to help him develop the water-drinking behavior, since the only fluids he would drink at present were limited amounts of cola and beer. Since this patient liked attention from the staff and his fellow patients, the plan was to reinforce each time he asked for water during the daytime with timer alarm, set off by the staff. This alerted patients and staff to start acclaiming our patient as a jolly good fellow. All the time that the patient was actually drinking water the staff and patients would clap their hands in applause. His water intake was charted on the wall graph, and each time he emptied his pitcher of water he was given a paper noise maker to blow, and the staff set off the timer alarm. The shaping process was to get the patient to perform the first step in drinking-water behavior, that of asking for water, a behavior that had not been in his repertoire. After this step was shaped, the rest of the process was to increase the water-drinking behavior with positive reinforcement, a process discussed in Chapter 5.

Fortunately, the water-drinking behavior was well established before satiation for the game on the part of the patient and others set in. Natural reinforcers, such as weight stabilization and the good systemic feeling from adequate fluid intake, became effective; the water-drinking game was no longer necessary.

The next patient problem is one that you have identified while being the nurse in charge in a nursing home. Your 80-year-old patient, Mrs. Black, is a shy grandmother whose family has had to move out of town for a year. She misses her relatives but is too shy to join the group activities. You are concerned because she sits quietly alone in her room for longer and longer periods of the day. You, your patient, and the consultant physical therapist develop a shaping plan toward group exercise. There are group exercise sessions twice a day in the activity room, but your patient will watch from her wheelchair occasionally and never join in. The shaping plan is to teach the exercises to your patient in the privacy of her room. The first exercise is taught, and when Mrs. Black has completed it, you write a letter for her to her grandson. The next day you repeat the process but ask her to join the group for just that exercise. When she succeeds in completing that first exercise with the group, you go back to her room with her and write a letter for her to her daughter. The next day you teach Mrs. Black another exercise and ask a volunteer to share a letter from Mrs. Black's granddaughter and to help her write an answer. The following day you, the volunteer, and Mrs. Black rehearse the two exercises in her room and then join the group for those exercises. The volunteer takes your patient back to her room to help her with another letter. The next day after learning the third and fourth exercises, Mrs. Black asks to stay for the whole group exercise session; she thinks she can catch on to what they are doing. Mrs. Black enjoys the group session and goes to the room of Mrs. White, her exercise partner, for the purpose of seeing pictures of Mrs. White's grandchildren. The natural reinforcers of solidarity and friendship have become effective. Your staff has perhaps prevented one of the saddest byproducts of untreated retreat from society; namely, isolation or social deprivation.

Another example of shaping a behavior is helping an elderly person put on his elastic bandage for the purpose of facilitating venous return. This 85-year-old gentleman, Mr. Smith, needs to put this elastic bandage wrap onto his left leg each morning and rewrap it every afternoon; he does not wear it at night. His daughter-in-law used to do this task for him, but she has moved away. You, as a visiting nurse, have taught your home health aide how to help patients to shape in this procedure. This is another situation where it is necessary to finish the procedure; so instead of allowing your patient to become discouraged by his doing a sloppy job, you program small approximations of the completed task and have the aide help Mr. Smith finish the whole task properly. Your aide may have to spend several minutes in bandage rolling and the first step of anchoring the bandage before any more steps can be learned. She gives him praise for each small step completed. The aide has an effective reinforcer; when the bandaging session is completed, a hot lunch is ready for Mr. Smith. He likes to have her eat her sack lunch with him. The one day he refuses to complete his bandaging task, the aide does not scold, but she does not stay to eat with him. She leaves his lunch ready for him to eat alone. The next session he completes his task quickly, and there is time for a leisurely lunch and conversation. When Mr. Smith learns to do his leg wrapping, the aide has more time to help him start a window-box tomato garden. Later, he has time to play a game of double solitaire with his neighbor instead of spending much of the afternoon leg-wrapping. The natural reinforcers are taking over, and the self-care leg-wrapping continues.

The intensive care ward also can use shaping techniques in behavior modification. After surgery your patient needs to help himself as much as possible for the purpose of promoting circulation and preventing the results of the disuse syndrome, such as contractures and isolation deprivation. You protect your intensive care patient from severe fatigue; you arrange rest periods during his care, when no team member disturbs the patient unless there is an emergency. Yet, although he regularly has time out from the intensive and varied stimulation of care, he still may become a passive recipient; satiation of stimulation may extinguish his paying attention to the world around him; and he may appear confused. You attempt to get him involved in his care by shaping his turning-in-bed behavior. Instead of two nurses quickly turning him without his participation, you add the procedure of supporting his hand and arm over to the side rail toward which he is turning. When he touches the rail you pat him and praise him. Your team does not have time to stand and wait for the patient; the shaping is included as the patient is turned. You praise your patient for grasping the rail, pulling on the rail, and finally initiating the pulling on the rail when you give him a cue that it is time to turn. You continue the shaping as you teach him the steps of turning his lower extremities. You teach him how to push himself up in bed. He learns bed mobility and is rewarded for it. This may help to prevent contractures, decubiti, stasis pneumonia, and constipation. Listening to and responding to the team during these activities may help him stay oriented to time, place, and person. It is a real time to turn in bed; you are a real person as he responds to your teaching, and you and he are both in a real hospital where you and the other members of the health care team treat him as an individual who can respond to a positive reinforcer. He is someone to interact with as well as to care for physically.

Ambulation is another area of patient teaching where you can use shaping techniques effectively. Each step from sitting balance, standing balance, wheelchair transfer, wheelchair ambulation, and finally to walking ambulation has several minor steps or behaviors that need to be reinforced before the terminal target behavior, walking, can be reached for some patients. The process of locking wheelchair brakes, putting feet on the floor, sliding forward, and standing erect may call for careful reinforcement for each step in each task.

It is prudent for you to take advantage of all the mechanisms available to help you and your patient during the learning process. You may be able to help the stroke patient perform these tasks in the preparation-for-walking series but find that the patient cannot remember to include all the steps consistently. The patient may forget to lock the brakes one day or forget to take his or her foot off the footrest the next day. You may fashion a cue card in the form of printed tasks on a tape placed on the arm of your patient's wheelchair. Now the patient can rehearse the correct order of the tasks that have been shaped. Again, the patient may learn by repetition and success the order in which the tasks should be performed and may no longer need the cue tape. Similarly, you may help another patient shape walking behavior by helping him or her to perform a series of approximations of the terminal behavior. The patient may practice standing balance in the parallel bars and progress to a walker or to a four-footed cane; then may finally walk without any assistive device. The patient will progress faster if each minor step is successfully learned by shaping rather than if he or she becomes anxious because of not knowing how to do the task.

You may have an opportunity to make the shaping process much easier if the staff has written a complete nursing history. For example, a patient's wife has been asked to take her husband's blood pressure every day and to bring the record to the physician at the next clinic visit. You have rechecked the family interview at the time of admission and find that the nurse recorded the wife's statement as to how difficult it is for her to do things well enough to earn her husband's approval. The wife is encouraged to learn the procedure in very small steps, and she has an opportunity to practice on nurses and orderlies until you are certain that she can perform the terminal behavior expertly. You check her accuracy by utilizing a stethoscope with a double earpiece set, which allows you to hear the same sounds she hears. She tells you she is ready to take her husband's blood pressure and asks you to check her accuracy with the instructor's stethoscope. Her husband is pleased that his wife's measurements correspond with yours. She is grateful to have learned the procedure by successful steps instead of by fear of failure.

It is important when shaping behavior that you set up the training environment in a manner that allows some probability that a successful unit of behavior will occur. If you are shaping self-feeding behavior in a stroke patient or in a severely ill patient, you should clear the area of distractions and use any devices by which to make the task easier. If the plate slides, you can use a suction pad or a wet cloth to help the patient have some chance for success. The patient should be able to see the right side of the tray (that is, where the food should be), and the units of behavior being practiced should be short so that the positive reinforcement of warm food occurs instead of an aversive stimulus, cold food.

It is important for the nursing staff to understand the shaping technique because the team may depend on the nurses to help another team member control the reinforcers and indirectly to help the patient succeed in the shaping process. For example, some patients may have an abnormal behavior, such as an abnormal gait, that they wish to change. The physician may become the reinforcer and attend to the patient only after the gradual shaping step for the day has been performed. This process may occur only in the physical therapy department at a specific time, thus allowing the physician an opportunity to schedule time for the purpose of being available to reinforce the progress consistently. To control the contingency of the physician reinforcing successful behavior and to prevent the possibility of the abnormal gait being reinforced, the team may agree to watch carefully that the patient ambulates by wheelchair at all other times. This process is set up by means of a verbal treatment contract with the patient and the team, as has been mentioned in preceding chapters. The patient will need the support of the whole team. If the patient sees the team take this treatment contract seriously, he or she will be less inclined to be embarassed by possible ridicule from teasing patients. The nurses help the patient by being socially nonresponsive to any patients who are teasing the patient. The nurses will find ways to divert the activities away from paying attention to the wheelchair behavior of the patient. They will turn attention to the wall graph depicting progress in physical therapy and to sharing the successful progress reports with the patient and friends. The wheelchair ambulation part of the program will be played down because the patient might be embarrassed. The shaping program will continue until the patient is ambulating normally outside the parallel bars. All the time that this shaping process is going on, the team must be exploring methods by which the patient will come in contact with reinforcers to continue normal walking after discharge. This subject is covered in Chapter 9.

PRACTICE PROBLEMS

As stated at the beginning of this chapter, shaping is the technique used to develop a behavior that has a rate close to zero or that happens at random. Shaping is based on reinforcing nearer and nearer approximations of the target behavior with emphasis on planning small enough steps to ensure a very high probability of frequent reinforcement. To test the technique, evaluate the following examples:

1. A teenaged leukemia patient is home after having a bone marrow transplant. He had been very ill in the hospital and finds it difficult to get back to working on his lessons, even though he was used to studying 3 hours after dinner before he became ill. He has asked his visiting nurse, whose attention he likes, to help him get started again. Which beginning plan do you think is most likely to succeed?

    Plan A: The nurse selects a morning half hour when she thinks her patient will be the most comfortable and rested; sees that all his school supplies are handy; and tells him she will be back in 30 minutes to hear what he has learned.

    Plan B: The nurse selects a morning half hour when she thinks her patient will be the most comfortable and rested; sees that all his school supplies are handy; and starts asking him questions about the subject he is studying, which he can answer already or quickly look up. She stays with him and praises highly every time he comes up with the right answer.

    Plan B is most likely to succeed because the example information indicated that the patient had not been able to start himself and was needing to shape in some start-to-study behaviors. The nurse set up opportunities for the patient to be reinforced immediately after each approximation of start-to-study behavior before a conflicting response could intervene, such as "reading-the-funnies-first." In Plan A there was no program for shaping or reinforcing the start-to-study behavior; it was left to chance. It is likely that the nurse will be able to judge the patient's fatigue threshold and will be able to plan with him realistic increments of study time. As the patient increases his study time without fatigue, the nurse will lean out the reinforcement schedule.

2. Mrs. Taylor, a 55-year-old housewife, brings her 65-year-old husband home from the hospital after major surgery complicated by thrombophebitis. He has been in the hospital 5 weeks and is weak, overweight, and apathetic. Mrs. Taylor had

spoken with the surgeon about her husband's occasional inability to have an erection during intercourse and was advised that the surgery should not interfere; in fact, things should be better because her husband no longer had hip or back pain. The physician also advised her to keep attempting intercourse even though her husband was apathetic.

Mrs. Taylor's visiting nurse, Mary Field, was helping her teach her 20-year-old son how to manage his insulin injections since he had just been diagnosed a diabetic, when Mrs. Taylor broke down in tears and asked the nurse to help her with her personal problem. Mrs. Taylor had already defined her target behaviors; she wanted to have intercourse with her husband twice a week. The Taylors had had no successes since Mr. Taylor's surgery 3 months previously. Mrs. Taylor described to the nurse that she had tried everything including candlelight dinners and the very best wine, but she thought Mr. Taylor was not caring enough about how she felt; he was still apathetic. Mary suggested to Mrs. Taylor that she was responsible for her own sexual pleasure and that she should plan to achieve it (Masters and Johnson, 1975).

Mary helped Mrs. Taylor understand that heavy dinners and no exercise could be negative factors, while exercise, light meals, and a small amount of wine in the evening might be positive factors toward her goal. In order to help Mrs. Taylor improve her sexual function, Mary set up a program with Mrs. Taylor which included daily praise over the telephone if Mrs. Taylor reported completing her program of:

   a.   Open communication with Mr. Taylor every day
   b.   Beginning exercise program with Mr. Taylor every day
   c.   Light meals with Mr. Taylor four times every day

After 2 weeks of success with the beginning program, Mary described to Mrs. Taylor how to utilize manual stimulation and hand cream lubrication to help Mr. Taylor attain and maintain an erection and attain coitus (Eisenberg and Rustad, 1975).

After 2 more weeks, the Taylors utilized the technique two times a week. Six weeks from the beginning of the program, manual stimulation was no longer necessary, and the Taylors elected to continue their twice-weekly schedule. In this case, the nurse reinforced Mrs. Taylor, but Mrs. Taylor did the shaping with Mr. Taylor.

SUMMARY

Shaping is the reinforcement of closer and closer approximations of the desired or target behavior. When starting the process, reinforce the approximation quickly before a conflicting response intervenes. Make each increment small, because a too-advanced step can prevent success from occurring, and the shaping process will be momentarily stopped. Know your patient well, because shaping is more effective if you can anticipate how large a step of progress he or she can handle with good chances of success.

8
PUNISHMENT

DEFINITION

Punishment, as that term is usually used, is rarely a treatment approach that health care professionals would want to consider or use. There are many obvious ethical and moral reasons why that is so, which need no further comment here. There are also a number of other disadvantages, which we shall mention, to the use of punishment. Before proceeding, however, let us consider more carefully just what punishment is and is not.

Strictly speaking, there are two concepts, or definitions, of punishment. One is the application of an aversive or noxious stimulus, as when a mother spanks a child or a supervisor openly and sharply berates an employee. That is the use of the term that we ordinarily think of, and that is the kind of punishment we think is rarely indicated in patient care methods.

The second way to define punishment is as the withdrawing of positive reinforcers, as when a mother lets her child no longer have candy if he or she displays tantrum behavior. The mother has withdrawn a reinforcer, candy, that may have been supporting tantrum behavior; or, more likely, withdrawal of the reinforcer could become an effective way of helping her child learn not to have temper tantrums by making that reinforcer contingent upon the child's engaging in nontantrum behavior. In either case, when the mother takes the candy away she is, in one sense of the term, punishing her child. She is at the same time creating conditions that will help her child to learn a better way of behaving.

Both definitions of punishment have the common characteristic of encouraging or causing the person to avoid the punishment by doing something else. If the mother spanks her child for tantrum behavior, she hopes the child will now avoid tantrum behavior because it leads to spanking. If the mother withdraws candy when the child has a tantrum, she hopes her child will now avoid tantrum behavior in order to avoid losing the candy. Punishment as an aversive stimulus suppresses but does not reduce behavior; and that kind of punishment also interferes with the nurse-patient relationship.

IMPLEMENTATION

The major effect of punishment is that it establishes aversive conditions that are avoided by any behavior of "doing something else"; it might even be the behavior of "holding still."

On the pediatric ward you may observe a healthier child pounding on a very weak child with his fist; as you come up to the children you will say, "Stop, Johnny." Johnny does not stop; you will hold his arm to prevent injury to the other child. Having his hand restrained even momentarily is an aversive stimulus to Johnny, yet this gives you time to allow the second child to escape and for you to start an activity that both children will enjoy.

Your pediatric patient may be about ready to pour orange juice over his head; your aversive "no" may give you time to get to the child's side and to praise him for pouring juice into himself instead of onto himself.

The graph in Figure 9 illustrates the progress of a 6-year-old boy whose negative behavior was interfering with his practicing self-care skills. Crying, biting, and spitting during practice time interfered with progress and gave little time to reinforce productive behavior. Time-out technique was instigated. This was a plan in which the child was removed from the scene of action to the quiet, neutral environment of his room. The toy box was removed at this time, and the nurse's soft comment was, "It is time to rest now." Thirty minutes later, and if there were no disruptive behaviors, the lad was brought out of his room, and a "new" day was started without comment. In this way the positive reinforcers, toys and attention from the staff, were withdrawn for short periods of time. In contrast, periods of effective behavior gave him access to staff reinforcement for more constructive efforts, such as smiling, talking appropriately, and productive play or work. The summary graph indicates the increased positive be-

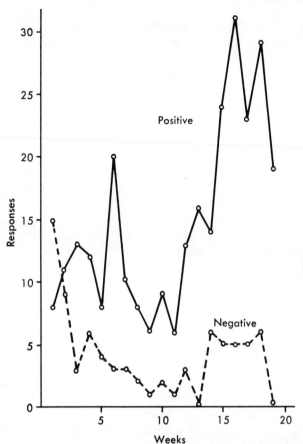

Figure 9. Increased positive units of behavior and decreased negative units of behavior by reinforcement. Units of behavior recorded in the nurses' daily charting.

haviors, which were counted from the nursing notes in a retroactive study. The process was difficult at first for the nurses because the child was cute and in need of help. Thus they were reluctant in the beginning to punish the boy. However, they stuck to the project, and their efforts were rewarded when their little patient used the toilet instead of diapers, dressed himself, and amused himself by making model cars.

The next example illustrates withdrawal of a positive reinforcer, although we could say that all that was done was to rearrange the timing of the positive reinforcer. Occasionally, you, the nursing team leader, may have difficulty identifying the need for a punishment technique. You may have a patient who has been willing to cooperate with a behavior modification program and has been active in planning the reinforcer for weight gain. Your patient, Mr. Fox, is in need of high-protein and high-caloric consumption in order to recover completely from surgery. You have identified the target behavior as eating all his meals, and you are measuring his progress on a daily weight graph, which he fills in. You and your team praise Mr. Fox for his weight gain, but you know from your experience that he is not progressing fast enough. You and your team review the behavior modification program, checking for possible mistakes in the system. You decide to keep a calorie count of intake for each meal; the dietary department is willing to note the calorie intake on the chart after each tray is returned to the pantry from Mr. Fox's room. The data indicate that the evening meal is the offender; he eats about half of the food sent to him for dinner. What is wrong? Is the food cold at that time of day, or is the menu less inviting at that time? Your evening nurse watches carefully what the situation is like during that meal. She finds an interesting phenomenon: one pretty little member of the team had not had the complete communication; she is the girl who delivers the tray. This young lady tells the nurse that she knows that Mr. Fox should eat, so when she finishes passing the trays, she goes back to Mr. Fox's bedside and coaxes him to eat a little something every night. Your system needs a slight revision; you explain the team's program to the tray girl, and withdraw her, the positive reinforcer, for Mr. Fox's "picking at his evening meal" behavior. Strictly speaking, it is true that you have punished Mr. Fox. You are careful, however, to reinforce the more desired behavior of eating by arranging for the girl to come back to chat with him if his evening meal is eaten. That is, you have withdrawn the reinforcer of the girl's attention from noneating behavior in order to help the patient to reduce that destructive behavior. But you have also attached the reinforcer to the constructive eating behavior. Mr. Fox is pleased that his weight gain has improved and that he is going home in 2 days.

The use of punishment just described is a helpful and essential part of good patient management. What it does is to let reinforcers become contingent upon desired target behaviors instead of either being noncontingent or being contingent upon undesired or self-defeating behaviors. Reinforcers are being put to work to help not hurt the patient.

Aversive stimuli may be aversive for some patients and not for others; employed carefully and sparingly, they can sometimes be useful toward fulfilling an important goal. You are the head nurse on an extended care unit, and you have to make a room assignment decision for an incoming 72-year-old male patient who is paralyzed on the left side. You know from your data base from the hospital that this patient needs to be out of his room most of the day and that he needs to socialize with other patients. You have two rooms available; one is a two-bed room with a patient who is going home tomorrow, and the other is a room whose occupant plays and listens to his loud music all day except rest time and bedtime. The music-loving patient will be going home in 4 days; you hope this will give you enough time to get your new patient involved in the social activity, but that it will not provide too much aversive stimulation to the point where he might want to "escape." Your program worked; your patient avoided the aversive stimulus, loud music, and was well acquainted with the facility and other residents before his roommate went home. His involvement in one special activity, socializing, was incompatible with staying in his room all day. One natural positive reinforcer, successful social activity, found in the environment had become effective.

Wenrich (1970) states that an aversive stimulus is any stimulus that an organism (if given the opportunity) will escape from, avoid, or terminate. These words describe physical or psychological pain or discomfort. Put yourself in this outpatient clinic nurse's place: you and your patient have a very difficult problem to solve. Your patient, 45-year-old Mrs. Graham, is 30 pounds overweight; she is ashamed, uncomfortable, sleepy, and has aching feet. She has seen her physician, and she has tried diet pills, special diets, and behavior modification programs using fines, rewards, and combinations of positive reinforcers and aversive stimuli; but she can only hold the line for over a year; she cannot seem to lose any more pounds. Mrs. Graham has a supportive family, and the family members have cooperated with every weight-loss plan that has been tried; but no lasting success has evolved. You are concerned for your patient because she expresses feelings of hopelessness. You know that behavior can usually be modified if you have control over a potent reinforcer. What is that reinforcer for Mrs. Graham? High-frequency behavior is often a cue to or is itself a potent reinforcer. You observe Mrs. Graham very carefully as you prepare your data base, and you ask her and her family what things does she do most often, and what and whom does she most often talk about? One person comes up high on everyone's list: her oldest son, who is a student and lives away from home. He has done exceptionally well in all areas that she values, and she is very proud of him. She also feels that his respect for her is less, since she has been unable to use self-control in her eating behavior. He is accessible because he usually comes home for Sunday dinners. All the family members agree to the trial of 6 months, during which the oldest son will visit when his mother is home only if she has lost an additional pound that week and not until the quota of 1 pound lost per week is met on a cumulative basis. If his mother loses 1 pound in 1 week, the son visits; if she fails the next week to lose and does not gain, she must have lost 2 pounds to earn the next week's visit. The family members keep the weight record on the refrigerator door; the father supervises the weekly weigh-in, and he joins the program, too, because he is overweight. But the major program is centered on Mrs. Graham's avoiding the loss of not hearing from or not seeing her son. This program works for Mrs. Graham this time, even though there are some plateaus as the weight loss levels out sometimes for 3 weeks in a row. Mrs. Graham cannot cheat on the program; she cannot play the game this week and then skip a week. You and the whole family have found a potent reinforcer, and you have the reinforcer under control.

It could be argued that in this example, punishment was not involved, that the real program was shaping, using a reward, the son's visit. Your patient describes that she worked hard to avoid the possibility of the sight of the empty chair at Sunday dinner. Certainly the Sunday visits were reinforcing in the initial phases of the program, but also some natural, unprogrammed reinforcers began to appear. Mrs. Graham's clothes felt more comfortable; other clothes began to fit; she had more energy from the well-balanced diet; her feet felt good again; and the whole family had more fun and came home more with friends because Mrs. Graham had become herself again. Skiing and playing basketball with her younger sons took over much of the eating and snacking time. Mrs. Graham was happy to have her son's respect again, but she did not need the weekly visits as the family became more and more active and independent. You close the case because Mrs. Graham does not feel the need to come to clinic. In passing, we should note that this example is a particularly good illustration of how generalization may work. The topic of generalization is discussed in the next chapter, and we shall refer back to this case in that context.

In the following example you are a rehabilitation nurse at the point where the rehabilitation team faces a patient's problem that demonstrates many of the concepts discussed so far. The patient's problem could be called avoidance behavior conditioned by an aversive stimulus, the husband's rejection. Mrs. Ex, a 43-year-old housewife, is doing something to postpone or prevent pending adversity. She comes to the medical rehabilitation center seriously ill with anorexia nervosa, a chronic failure to eat. She weighs 63 pounds, and there are doubts as to her potential for survival. Her weight has been declining slowly over a 5-year period, from an estimated normal weight of 113 pounds. The medical service of a teaching hospital has referred her to the center because the numerous diagnostic and therapeutic procedures, both medical and psychiatric, have not reversed the weight loss process.

Behavioral analysis has been carried out by direct observation and by interview with her, her husband, and her 18-year-old son. The couple had been active in church work and community work together, but finally the husband had expressed a desire to marry someone else since the patient continually did housework after her husband's bedtime and before he awoke in the morning. The husband had contracted to postpone divorce until his wife was no longer critically ill. Mrs. Ex has had considerable attention from her family and friends and from medical staff because of her failure to eat. The target behavior to increase is eating. In other circumstances efforts would likely have been made to improve sexual relations in the marriage. In this instance, however, legal termination of the marriage was a certainty at the end of Mrs. Ex's medical crisis; in fact, actual termination had been effected for several years. Therefore, no commitment was made to salvage the marriage.

Your nursing team observes and charts two high-frequency behaviors identified on the ward; namely, chatting with the staff and being busy with personal tasks and jigsaw puzzles. You join the other rehabilitation team members in setting a program using attention from staff members as the reinforcer. The target behavior, eating, is measured by calorie intake and the resultant weight status, using standard conditions of calorie measurement and weight measurement. Mrs. Ex is provided with a weight progress graph, which is put on her wall. The entire staff praises her for weight gain, and all members are socially nonresponsive to failures to gain. You remind the new nurses to continue to chart the patient's high-frequency behaviors. Several days later the graph shows only a minimal weight gain, indicating that attention from the staff is a low-power reinforcer. The program is changed by the team, and activity is designated as the reinforcer for eating and weight gain. Three schedules of activity are written on a chart for Mrs. Ex's bulletin board: (A) no visitors; confinement to her room; no projects such as sewing, crocheting, or puzzles in the room; and no occupational therapy projects; (B) 1 hour of occupational therapy 2 times a day and 1 hour in the evening feeding severely disabled patients (if desired); (C) unlimited activity in occupational therapy, helping on the ward any time, and unlimited visiting hours. You have Mrs. Ex as your one-to-one patient, along with your usual assignment of 5 other patients. You come 10 minutes early every day, not to check on the patient's honor system of weighing-in, but to be certain that the ward scales are available and that Mrs. Ex has an opportunity to weigh-in each morning under standard conditions before breakfast. Another nurse does this for you on your days off because you often help her with details in caring for her one-to-one patient. The scales must be ready every morning, because under the new plan your patient needs to compare each morning's weight against her average weight attained the week before. The result of the comparison determines which schedule Mrs. Ex will be on each day: schedule A if she loses or only maintains her weight, schedule B if she increases her weight up to 2 pounds, schedule C if she increases her weight by more than 2 pounds. Proper diet is maintained, because schedules B and C do not go into effect unless Mrs. Ex eats the carefully planned meals the day before. Mrs. Ex enjoys feeding patients, and you program these experiences with patients who you judge will accept Mrs. Ex and will, by their response, keep this activity a rewarding one for both her and them. The physicians, therapists, nurses, and other members of the team continue to praise Mrs. Ex when she is seen working on some project out of her room. The psychologists are helpful to you as they give you feedback as to her progress in her short daily conferences with them. She has an opportunity to plan for her future, and it is reinforcing for you and the nursing staff to see her progress from 66 to 88 pounds in a little over 9 weeks.

It is particularly reinforcing for you to know that your patient leaves the hospital rehabilitation center to engage in full-time employment. Follow-up is important for your staff, and particularly for the new staff; they want to know how your patient is doing as time progresses after discharge. Follow-up is equally important for the patient while the natural reinforcers have time to materialize. Mrs. Ex maintains her weight while she is on a 6-week outpatient program. Fourteen months later at your weekly ward "milieu" meeting, you hear from the psychologist that Mrs. Ex has maintained her weight at 85 pounds and is doing nicely in spite of the fact that the legal divorce has been finalized. Three years later she is still doing well. The natural reinforcers are effective and increasing; new friends have been made, and her old friends from her church are again asking her to join them for lunch, since they no longer have to devote the lunch hour to her previous noneating behavior. In summary, her behavior changed while she was on a program that, first, withdrew positive reinforcers, activities, when noneating behavior occurred and that, second, added those same positive reinforcers when eating behavior occurred. Fortunately, natural reinforcers were available to maintain the target behavior—yet another example of generalization, a concept that is discussed in Chapter 9.

Escape from an aversive stimulus often causes a behavior to increase rapidly for a short period of time during which the nurse can set up a behavioral change system engineered for more lasting results and more pleasant implementation. For example, a 6-year-old boy is dehydrated and must take fluids orally or be subjected to another intravenous infusion. He promises that he will drink ample fluids if he can escape from the intravenous infusion. You know that he means what he says, but you also know that he drinks well for a while and then stops trying, which means a repetition of the whole cycle plus much frustration on the part of both the patient and the staff. This time you plan a contract with your patient. For every glass of fluid he drinks, he gets to have his miniature racer moved up the track on his bulletin board 1 inch; and when the racer reaches the top of the bulletin board, he gets a Popsicle. There is another stipulation in the contract; first, to escape from the needle he must drink four glasses of water to get his racer out of the "pit" and onto the bulletin board race track. The contract works, and he has had enough fluids to allow him time to play a game with his miniature racer. From day to day you may vary the game. One day you may set up a double track and two cars, letting him manipulate a race between two favorite doctors or his dad and his doctor. The probability is that the reinforcer will be strengthened as more and more staff are aware of the race and add their attention to his successful fluid-drinking behavior.

An example of escape from an aversive stimulus is the case of the adult patient who has been warned by his physician to stop smoking or to expect further pulmonary complications. Mr. Stack enlists your help by saying, "I wish someone would help me quit smoking instead of everyone telling me to quit smoking." You tell him you might be able to help him, but it will take some effort on his part, and you want to confer with him and the whole treatment team about your plan. On rounds the next day you suggest a behavioral change contract; it is a little unorthodox, and you have to give everyone time to discuss the possible pros and cons. The patient is enthusiastic for trial, and the team agrees to do the following: draw $50.00 of Mr. Stack's money out of the hospital safe and give it to his wife that evening to take home and put in a safe place; make a sign, to be put onto Mr. Stack's bulletin board, which reads, "I will pay the first person who catches me smoking a reward, $50.00, payable within 24 hours after the happening," signed George Stack and witnessed by Mrs. Stack; and also place a graph on the same bulletin board, which will indicate each 8 hours that Mr. Stack is not found to be smoking. You are using punishment, but only with his full consent and participation. You and your staff pay attention to Mr. Stack's graph and praise him as the line moves up every 8 hours; obviously you do not have to program monitors to check on the smoking or not-smoking behaviors. Your patient is discharged in 2 weeks with his $50.00 intact and with no cigarrette breath; you help your patient plan for natural monitors, such as his neighbors, office friends, and relatives. Six months later you hear from Mrs. Stack that your discharged patient is still a nonsmoker and has escaped losing $50.00 each of those 6 months.

UNDESIRABLE CONSEQUENCES

Punishment is commonly used because the user is generally reinforced by an immediate reaction on the part of the recipient. There is little evidence that the effect is more than temporary, and there is considerable evidence that punishment makes people unhappy.

One desirable consequence of punishment is a conflict between the response that leads to punishment and the response that avoids it, "and which you desire to increase. A child may be punished for an unkept room and then makes his brothers uneasy when they visit his room and squash a precisely fluffed pillow. Punishment does not create a negative probability that a particular response will be made; it creates a positive probability that an incompatible behavior will occur (Skinner, 1953).

Another undesirable consequence from punishment is that it evokes reflexes of anxiety, fear, anger, or frustration. It is even more difficult when the behavior punished is a reflex and the individual being punished cannot come up with an immediate opposite behavior. One of the saddest situations in our culture is that a parent will punish a child for a misbehavior until he cries and then spank him until he stops crying.

Punishment through the use of aversive stimuli often slows or negates your relationship with the patient. Effective communication with your patient may be lost or impaired. The effectiveness of your attention and personal regard as a positive reinforcer will have been lost or reduced.

The use of punishment in the form of aversive stimulation (or threat to do so) is rarely indicated. That use of punishment can prove helpful only when the behavior to be changed is of very high frequency or of great strength. The example of Mr. Stack's smoking habit is a good illustration. Punishment, or threat of it, if the aversive stimulus is strong enough, can serve to interrupt a very high-strength behavior for a period of time until more control is gained. When threatened with the immediate loss of $50.00, Mr. Stack was able to inhibit the cigarette smoking for a number of days during which both the craving began to diminish and other reinforcers had time to take more effect. In such instances, as was done with Mr. Stack, the patient should be a full and willing partner to the contract.

ALTERNATIVES

A response can be weakened by means other than punishment. Punishable behavior may be changed if the *circumstances* that evoke the behavior are changed. The visiting nurse may help a grandfather to be welcome at the dinner table again by suggesting a plate guard to prevent his pushing his food onto the table cloth; or if he should go to a restaurant, a plate guard could be made by having someone butter his bread and invert it around the edge of his plate. *Satiation* can help weaken behavior that might ordinarily be punished. Some children are fascinated by the act of lighting matches and will wait until the mother is out of the house and then engage in match lighting on the sly. One mother purchased a large box of wooden matches and encouraged her little boy to strike as many matches as he wanted. One hundred matches later, satiation had resulted, and the transparent behavior on the sly was not in evidence again. The *natural maturation* of children often will serve as an alternative to punishment. The punishing routine of toilet training too early can be avoided by allowing a little longer time to pass. Another use of the passage of time with children's problems is to arrange for the objectionable behavior to be *forgotten*. However, this is usually a very slow process. Opportunities to practice the behavior should be avoided. A particularly unpleasant record may be forgotten if it is lost, and the constant behavior of playing that particular record may be postponed even to the extent that the name of the record is forgotten. This need not be punishment in the terms of destroying or hiding the record; mothers of some teenagers just learn not to help search.

Reinforcement of an *incompatible behavior* is often an effective technique in lieu of punishment. It is direct positive reinforcement of a desired behavior that cannot take place at the same time as the undesired behavior. You have a patient who sleeps poorly at night and naps often during the day; you keep your patient busy and awake during the day with interesting things to do instead of sending him back to bed continuously at night or giving him sleeping medication.

Another effective technique by which to avoid the complications of punishment by aversive stimulation is extinction; that is, withdrawal of reinforcers from the bad behavior. The process is simple only if you know what reinforces the behavior you want eliminated and if you have the control of the reinforcer. The abusive verbal behavior of a patient in a four-bed ward is reinforced by upsetting the nurses in front of the other patients. The nurses decide to pity this man instead of becoming angry; he no longer upsets them, and his abuse also stops.

PRACTICE PROBLEMS

1. What are some of the disadvantages of punishment?
   A. The effect is usually temporary.
   B. It can evoke a reflex (e.g., crying, fear, anger), which makes it more difficult for the subject to counter with a more acceptable behavior.
   C. It can negate you as a reinforcer.
   D. It makes people unhappy.
2. What are some alternatives to punishment?
   A. Punishable behavior may be changed if the *circumstances* that evoke the behavior are changed.
   B. *Satiation* can help weaken behavior which might ordinarily be punished.
   C. Passage of time.
   D. Reinforcement of an *incompatible behavior.*
3. Are the following incompatible behaviors?

A.	Sleeping in the daytime	Painting, pottery in the activity room in the daytime	Yes (the behaviors cannot be done simultaneously)
B.	Not wearing antiembolic stockings for each leg	Wearing antiembolic stockings for each leg	Yes

C. Refusing all your medications	Taking all your medications	Yes
D. Screaming	Singing a song	No (it is possible to scream words and a tune)
E. Whining about pain	Laughing about funny exercises	Yes
F. Wetting the bed	Utilizing the commode	Yes
G. Sitting in a chair alone	Walking outside with people	Yes

SUMMARY

Punishment may be thought of either as the onset of an aversive stimulus or as the withdrawal of positive reinforcement. Punishment by aversive stimulation is rarely indicated, and then, only when the patient is in full agreement. That use of punishment might prove helpful in situations of very high-strength or frequent behaviors. In such cases the aversive stimulus can be used in initial phases of a treatment program to interrupt or inhibit the behavior long enough for the patient to gain more control so that a positive reinforcement program can begin.

Punishment in the form of withdrawal of positive reinforcement means nothing more than that positive reinforcers will become contingent upon occurrence of the desired target behavior; that is, those reinforcers will not occur if the target behavior does not occur.

9
GENERALIZATION

DEFINITION

Generalization, as pointed out in the excellent paper by Baer and Wolf (1967), can be seen in three related ways. Basically, the term refers to the extent to which a behavior learned in one situation will spread or generalize to others. More specifically, we might say that generalization has occurred if the following occur. First, a behavior learned in one environment occurs in another environment. Examples of this form of generalization include the first grader who learns to read in school and begins to read also at home and the patient who learns to dress himself in the hospital and continues to do so at home. Second, a behavior occurring at one time continues to occur at later times; it endures. This form of generalization is virtually the same as the first. The only difference is that it refers to the behavior occurring across time whether or not the setting changes. Examples are the patient who learns to irrigate his catheter and continues to do so indefinitely into the future and the dieter who continues to diet for months and years. Third, a set of behaviors broadens to include an even wider set of related behaviors; it expands in scope. Generalization in this sense refers to changing more and more behavior. For example, a patient may learn to perform three of six possible ADLs, such as dressing, feeding, and grooming, and then go on to expand the number of ADLs he or she does, such as bathing, catheter care, and so on.

IMPORTANCE

Baer and Wolf (1967) define a problem for the technology of behavior modification. They call it achieving generality of behavioral change. The principles of behavior modification help us change behavior, but there is little point in doing so unless that change in behavior can be maintained in the individual's or the group's customary environment. That importance of generalization cannot be minimized, because much of the behavioral change engineered in the health care setting will fail in the home setting unless generalization occurs. For example, if a patient goes home and fails to practice the self-care he has demonstrated in the hospital, the family may become very depressed. The patient may even be abandoned by his family. On the other hand, if the expatient whips through his dressing activities so he will not miss the daily 10:00 AM to noon poker game with the senior citizens club members, then the family, the staff, and most important, the patient are all positively reinforced.

APPROACH
Direct programming

External control. The external approach to generalization is one direct method of programming the natural, outside-the-hospital environment to positively reinforce the behavior. Much of the nursing process in the practice of nursing today is problem identification and problem solving. The professional nurse spends more and more time in patient teaching, attempting to help the patient generalize good health management from the behaviors he or she has practiced in the hospital to the home and outside environment, such as outpatient clinic. One of the most important services consumers should be able to expect is that the experts in health care will help them prevent problems. For example, in the case of the patient with the new ileostomy, as described in Chapter 6, there is a potential problem. Patients know they should call for help when needed, but often they hesitate too long. The husband is home part of the time to reinforce his wife's success, but what happens if there is a beginning sign of skin breakdown near the stoma? Is she going to put off calling for help because it might go away and then she would not have bothered the clinic people whom she does not know? Or will she call the expert clinic nurse she knows, just as she calls the hospital expert now? Situations do occur where the patient puts off calling; and serious complications, such as a need for more surgery, may arise. Fortunately, the hospital nurse has introduced the patient to the outpatient clinic nurse, who gives the patient her phone number in writing and the hours of the day when she can be reached. The outpatient clinic nurse is also an expert in stomal care, and she shows the patient around the clinic. The clinic nurse is spending this time to get to know this patient for the purpose of helping her to feel free to call about the smallest concern, thus preventing a possible major problem of serious skin breakdown. The visiting nurse or a community ostomy center could offer opportunities for comparable contingencies to those in the original hospital setting, making it easy for the patient to call for help when she needs it. The husband must be informed regarding these possible consequences; then he can reinforce his wife's behavior, that of calling the right people for this service of prevention–a behavior generalized from hospital setting to outside the hospital setting. The physician is a potentially valuable reinforcer to calling the right people for help; his or her participation and support of the plans as they develop add strength to the response of calling the right people for help when in doubt.

Another possible problem is that the ileostomy patient might do very well with skin care and with the specifics of appliance care, but she may only do exactly what she has been taught and limit her scope regarding this area of her life to past information and calling for help when in doubt. Behaviors eventually reflect the reinforcers available, not the reinforcers that other behaviors meet. Before she leaves the hospital, other patients or ostomy society members can show her opportunities for continual resources of support and information. The nurse gives her an address of an excellent journal on the subject; the husband can again facilitate this plan to set up a source of continual health care maintenance ideas by paying for the subscription. When the patient sees how well other people manage their ileostomies, she can imitate these role models and benefit by their example. The nurse must be careful to program opportunities for excellent role models so that they can outweigh any random mediocre role models.

Self-control. With direct programming the same patient as in the example above develops a degree of self-determination, or self-control. She may decide when, where, and how often she will manipulate certain variables of her care. She may choose a course of action different from all her advice as she thinks out the solution to some problem. She controls herself just as someone else could control her behavior externally. She may avoid getting up early by doing her care in the evening; she has made the decision, but eventually it must be accounted for with variables external to herself. She may want to sleep in because her husband has time to be at home in the late evening only. As her strength improves, she has access to natural reinforcers, such as playing golf. She is especially careful about her care so that the ostomy will not interfere with her golf game; generalization has set in.

In Chapter 8 we pointed out the example of the reprogrammed family and environment of Mrs. Graham. Because of the temporary reprogramming of family interaction and the home environment, Mrs. Graham's weight decreased. At this time naturally occurring reinforcers became available. Mrs. Graham felt better; she was not ashamed to be seen in ski pants or slacks; and her noneating behaviors were increasing via sports and activities with her family. The family was careful that the "get started skiing" behavior was reinforced by scheduling an all-family ski trip for her first few trips back to the mountain.

Indirect programming

Trapping. The mouse trap example described by Baer and Wolf is a drastic but clear example of the trapping approach in generalization. They point out that the fatal experience for the mouse demonstrates a situation of generalization: the behavior change in the mouse is uniform across all environments; it has expanded in scope; in fact, it is a massive change for the mouse; and the change shall endure, unfortunately for the mouse. It has another feature: this massive and enduring behavioral change occured with minimal effort on the part of the behavioral engineer, the housewife. She set the trap, baited it with cheese, and waited for the mouse's entry response, which was identified by the snap of the trap. This trapping process was useful in her evaluation of the process because she did not have to catch and kill the mouse with her hands (Baer and Wolf, 1967).

Trapping or programming a behavioral change of a fourth-grade boy had generalization as the goal. Mike's primary teachers had shaped the behavior, reading, but his family and teachers were concerned that the behavior had not generalized: it was still confined to the classroom; it was limited to assigned reading; and it was not enduring. Playing baseball and dreaming about baseball were becoming incompatible behaviors with any kind of reading. What kind of mousetrap and what kind of entry response were needed for generalization? A neighbor boy—we shall call him Tom—unknowingly became the behavioral engineer. Tom was interested in building and launching model rockets; he let Mike watch and copy. The entry response was going next door to see what Tom was doing; the trap snapped shut because Mike began reading every model rocket catalog, newspaper events about rocket launchings, and began to make model rockets. His own peer group became interested, and the behavior generalized across environments and into the future as he moved with his reinforcing peer group. He experienced the satisfaction of learning something interesting, and he looked around for other interesting things to learn; his reading behavior expanded in scope. This was an indirect method of effecting generalization; Mike was merely "hooked up" to the natural reinforcers.

Baer and Wolf (1967) summarize one approach to the solution of achieving generalization of behavioral change by suggesting that the behavioral engineer develop an appreciation of what behavioral traps exist fort he changes that are desired and an appreciation of what the entry responses to behavioral traps might be. In the above example, Mike's big brother could have taken Mike over to Tom's house with him if the entry response had needed to be programmed.

Implementation examples

Unsupported behavior will extinguish over time. That is why generalization is important. To interrupt or prevent extinguishing, nurses support and contribute to parent groups and patient-alumni groups. For example, you may be the clinic nurse who helps parents of disabled children to know other parents in similar situations. You may have a list of parents who are willing to leave their phone numbers for other parents to call. They may form a nucleus of interested people who are able to reinforce each other when one of their group becomes weary of always having to be the natural reinforcer for her child who needs imaginative praise for his self-care activities. The entire group may program outside speakers who offer new information and who show the parents respect for the fine care they provide under difficult circumstances. You may be instrumental in bringing this group into contact with a funding organization that can help with special equipment or special camps for the children, or help in the home to facilitate a vacation for weary parents. You may be the only individual who praises a tired mother for finding a way just to get her child into the clinic on clinic days. You may be the only health care team member who is able to engender enough solidarity with a proud mother for you to learn that her family is really hungry. You have the opportunity to start the process of offering genuine support to this reinforcement-starved and food-starved family; perhaps your channel is an immediate call to the social worker. One of the real reinforcers for your nursing process is the satisfaction that you have helped alleviate the sparse reinforcement schedule of family members who must be potent and enthusiastic reinforcers for their children.

Nurses, because of their closeness to the individual human being as he or she works from sickness to wellness, have opportunity to be richly reinforced by behaviors of self-help. It is reinforcing for you, the teacher, to see that the patient has learned behaviors of self-help by actual performance of the tasks. It is difficult for you when your patient returns with a decubital ulcer when you know he knows how to prevent them. All that teaching of skin care, skin checks with the hand mirror, turning, bed positioning, wheelchair push-ups, and so on (if he is an alumnus from a spinal cord injury program), all seem pointless, and the reinforcement schedule for you is about zero at the moment. You and your colleagues across the nation have heard all the reasons why decubiti occur, but you know that in this case the behaviors that prevent decubiti did not happen consistently. Why was there no effective generalization of careful decubiti prevention behavior? What happened to the elements necessary for generalization? You analyze the report from your patient. You learn that all went well until he took a trip to Mexico with his friends; he was not very careful then. The contingencies operating in one environment were not comparable to the contingencies operating in the Mexican trip environment. The friends, the peer group, were different and did not reinforce "be careful of your skin" behaviors. In fact, he was in the car for very long periods of time, with no room to do push-ups.

What can you do about all this? You can avoid reinforcing the behavior by giving him a "homecoming" welcome or by giving him negative attention in the form of lectures or disgust. You can continue to reinforce his good skin care behavior when it occurs and share with the team the information he has given you about the trip to Mexico. There are decisions to be made and proposed plans to evaluate, each being weighed against the likelihood of generalization being effective when he leaves the hospital this time. The team decides that an active peer group that reinforces careful skin care behavior is essential. This is not easy to come by for many patients. The organized larger groups are often avoided by patients, but that is where the members of the team start. They may find some individuals who can help your mutual patient begin to build some productive peer relationships. This is why your nursing staff continue to support organizations and patient-alumni groups who might be able to help. As in any group chosen to reinforce well-behavior and self-care, the role models should be carefully selected. Sometimes there is a better supply of good role models than at other times, but your staff continue to keep in touch with their productive graduates, and they always make them welcome on the nursing unit. The less successful graduates are always welcome, but they are not invited to serve as good skin care role models. It is interesting to note that productive patients with spinal cord injuries are usually careful about decubiti prevention; they cannot afford to be hospitalized and lose all that time.

If you are caring for acutely ill patients, you have little time for extensive shaping of your patients' behavior; and although you have less time to try to prepare the outside environment for the purpose of generalization of behaviors learned in the hospital, you have some opportunity to do so. You have brief access to the families in some instances, but at other times the family stay close by the patient. Here you can share with the family what the visiting nurse should be able to do in assisting them to find reinforcers for good health care at home that are similar to those being used in the hospital.

Let us say you are on a busy medical floor, and your elderly patient was admitted with the diagnosis of diabetic coma caused by failure to manage her medications. There is no space for her to live in the home of her children; she was unsafe with her medications when she was living alone. Can she remain in her home? You cannot stop with your duties now, but you can give the family the social worker's number and the number of the appropriate visiting nurse. If natural reinforcers cannot be utilized to help this patient learn to be more careful with her medicine, perhaps the home environment can be reprogrammed for a little more support. Perhaps neighbors and the visiting nurse, home health aide, and the family can program themselves to monitor the medicines; in addition, this team in the home environment can program a reinforcing day each day in order to prevent further isolation deprivation and confusion. You will most likely interest the physician and the psychologist, if they are available, in helping to support the program.

If, on the other hand, this same patient seemed to you to be able to learn her medication routine, you can set up a calendar charting sheet for her to check off as she gives herself her medication; she practices this task in the hospital. You may then need minimal monitoring in the home by the visiting nurse, who would be checking on the patient's general health, daily activities, medication taking, and other needs, such as transportation to the senior citizens center, where the patient can be reinforced by her peer group for good personal care.

In comprehensive rehabilitation centers the health care team is made up of many members, including the physiatrist, who is the physician in charge, the psychologist, the social worker, the rehabilitation nurse, the occupational therapist, the speech pathologist, the physical therapist, the vocational counselor, the prosthetist-orthotist, the recreational therapist, and many other resource people from the community. All these people are engaged in the activity of helping the most important person on the team, the patient, to gain function. This team is effective in helping many patients return to their homes, but occasionally there is no place for an elderly grandmother to go but to an extended care facility or to a nursing home. What can the team do for this patient after the team members have helped her regain as much function as possible? A site visit to the nursing home by the rehabilitation nurse can facilitate communication and planning for the daily living of this patient. The patient has been well taught by her occupational therapist, and she can perform her ADLs with some skill; now the concern is that she have opportunity to use these skills in the environment of the nursing home. It is important for this poststroke patient to feel useful, and it is important that the environment reinforce her skills. More and more nursing homes are attempting to prevent confusion from stimulus deprivation; they are willing to try to find ways to prevent their residents from becoming confused, depressed, and bed-bound.

Let us say that you are making the site visit, and Mrs. Green, your patient, is coming with you. Since Mrs. Green has no family in the state, you will help her get her things into the nursing home. The nurses know you are coming, and you have planned to arrive at the time the residents and nurses have coffee together in the morning. Mrs. Green is given a special welcome and has opportunity to meet her day nurse aide and several residents. Mrs. Green is taken on a tour of the nursing home while you give your report to the charge nurse. In the course of the discussion you learn that the volunteer in the activity room has an electric frying pan, which is used for making popcorn on special occasions. At your suggestion she is willing to allow Mrs. Green to use the pan for making cookies for the party coming up in 2 days. You are pleased that this facility has found a way for Mrs. Green to transfer a special activity from her first environment to the second. Mrs. Green has taken your suggestion to call a member of her church group; a member will visit her Sunday. You will make a follow-up call in 2 weeks, and you hope to see Mrs. Green reinforced by the natural reinforcers in the facility, sociable human beings and purposeful activities. You have a hunch that you may be asked to try to find a group of volunteers to help supply

Mrs. Green with frozen cookie dough, since the activity room has some limitations. This task is becoming less and less difficult, since some of the girls' groups have a Foster Granddaughter program where they "adopt" a grandfather or grandmother for 6 months for their service projects.

For the purposes of generalization in behavior modification, natural reinforcers are an ideal situation; but sometimes we have to settle for a little less. You are charge nurse in a nursing home, and you have attempted to enrich the environment of stimulation by supporting a program of Foster Grandparents. It would be better if your residents had their own grandchildren to visit and to feel wanted by them, but you have one alternative. You have programmed a trip twice a week to the home for retarded children. You or the social workers must do the driving, but it is well worth it to see two groups of people in need find satisfaction through the project. The self-dressing behavior that the patients learned at the rehabilitation center is reinforced by getting to go help the children after these "grandparents" have dressed themselves in the morning.

At present there are relatively few occasions when a hospital nurse can become involved in helping set up home environment to have the same reinforcers as those programmed during the treatment phase in the hospital; the nurse works through a direct programmer, such as the visiting nurse or a member of the family. It is not unusual for the professional nurse to spend considerable time with the family member or attendant who will be the nearest human reinforcer to the patient. Occasionally, the nurse is asked to facilitate special opportunities for family teaching. One case involved a young man who had recently become quadriplegic from poliomyelitis. Oxygen support was being administered through his tracheostomy. His young wife was delivered of their first child in the same hospital; she then proceeded to make plans to move the family to Montana via station wagon. The nurse attempted to simulate environment number two by moving a cot and crib into the patient's room. Then the shaping began as the young wife learned the approximation leading to the care of quadriplegic husband and a newborn infant. Reinforcing feedback arrived to the effect that the family made the trip safely with the help of portable oxygen and the learning process through shaping at the hospital. The direct-care environments were similar enough to expect generalization, and the natural reinforcers in their own home away from the big city were at that time maintaining the behaviors learned.

More and more we are learning to take advantage of the principles of behavior modification. It is probably prudent to continue to find ways to change the behavior of chronically disabled patients because our population is made up of so many more elderly people and because the automobile continues to increase the rate of serious injury. One concept that is continually in clearer view is that more time should be spent reprogramming the home environment than in the hospital environment. On a rehabilitation ward there used to be a system that called for certain independent behaviors from the paraplegic patients before they could go home on pass. For example, young Mrs. Snow was graduated to the "independent" private room with shower. In this room she was on her own: no services were offered except housekeeping; her meals were in the dining room; and there was no help from nursing service except to restock her supply shelf when she asked. The reasoning behind this do-it-yourself room was logical. It was believed that if Mrs. Snow rehearsed her turning by setting her own alarm clock, she would be better able to perform these tasks at home. She had a long list of important activities of daily living; a high percentage of the items were to be completed each day. If she succeeded for 4 days, she was to have her pass for a weekend at home. Mrs. Snow turned herself faithfully, and completed all her tasks. The staff and patient were pleased to see her leave the ward for the weekend, but they were concerned when they heard her description of her holiday: "Oh, I just slept and rested!"

The problem is not in the logic of rehearsing tasks to build up skill in self-care; rather the problem is the change in reinforcers between the hospital environment and the home environment. Escape in the example above was the patient's response to the busy hospital schedule, which could have been labeled an aversive stimulus. At home there was a sparse reinforcement schedule to do anything, so doing nothing did not make Mrs. Snow miss anything. The plan continued, but it was modified. The next weekend when she went home, she took her ADL checklist with her. The reinforcement was as follows: list completed meant dinner out with her husband; list not completed meant that her husband would bring her back to the hospital Saturday evening. Mrs. Snow returned Sunday, reporting a very good time. The process worked better because the second environment had a stronger reinforcer, and the husband was actively involved and moved across environments.

The closer you can keep the patient to the home environment, and the stronger you can make the home reinforcers, the more likely is the successful generalization of behaviors learned in the hospital. This is why nurses play an important role in making it possible and pleasant for the patient's family to visit. If for some reason the family members are overprotective, you should not exclude them; you will not have a better opportunity to reinforce them for reinforcing independence in the patient. You will not be able to change their behavior if you exclude them or make them uncomfortable. You may find yourself reprogramming patient, staff, and family; but if it leads to the patient's self-respect, your reprogramming will usually be right.

PRACTICE PROBLEMS

Evaluate each of the following examples regarding generalized behavior:

1. The mother worked hard at her sewing because her daughters praised her, and the family had money for vacations from the savings she could set aside from the clothing budget. (The mother's behavior is generalized because it is hooked up to two natural reinforcers, daughters' praise and family vacations. She would probably sew even if the family moved, and the behavior is likely to endure as long as the daughters praise her and her efforts help generate family vacations.)

2. The nurse works overtime without pay at least twice a week. (The nurse's behavior is generalized because she works overtime no matter what shift she works and this behavior has endured for 2 years. Analysis indicates that this primary nurse is hooked on the natural reinforcers of patient, family, peer, and hierarchical praise for her comprehensive follow-through of nursing care and planning. It is also likely that she will be promoted while staying in her present type of work and preferred geographical location.)

3. The high-level quadriplegic patient is going to live by himself in an apartment and is certain he will keep up his positioning and skin care as well as he has done it in the hospital. (It is unlikely that this newly learned skin care behavior will generalize because the patient has no natural reinforcers to keep those difficult independent behaviors going. He may take the advice of the health care team and live with his family until he has finished learning his job skills and can pay attendant care. He possibly could generalize his skin care by keeping track of what the attendent does to protect the skin from decubiti. The natural reinforcers might be staying out of the hospital by checking his skin care. Staying out of the hospital would make it possible for him to hold his job and retain the new friends he has made. Then checking-on-skin-care behavior is likely to generalize and to endure.)

SUMMARY

Approaches or strategies to effecting generalization may be described as (1) direct programming of the natural environment to positively reinforce behavior, as described under external control and self-control, or (2) indirect trapping, where the subject is hooked up to a natural reinforcer, which in turn leads to many other natural reinforcers, which increase the probability that the behavioral change will endure. Baer and Wolf (1967) suggest that changed behavior, if truly generalized, should manifest itself in all environments, should expand in detail and scope, and should endure.

10
SYSTEM PLANNING

In the preceding chapters we have described the behavior analysis process as a tool that aids in solving certain problems confronting the patient and the other members of the health care team. In the next three chapters we describe three steps toward the *utilization* of this behavior analysis tool; namely, system planning, system implementation, and system evaluation. A facilitating system, problem-oriented charting, is illustrated in Chapter 12.

DEFINITIONS

A *process* is a logical and orderly way of doing something, a method, such as the helping process, the nursing process, and the behavior analysis process. A *system* is a carefully developed, relatively complex method, such as the utilization of the behavior analysis process within a health care facility or agency. *Problem-oriented charting* is a recording system, which, if done properly, facilitates the prudent utilization of most health care tools (Weed, 1969). This recording system requires the documentation of the patient's problems, plans for management of each problem, and the measurement of the extent of the predicted goal attainment.

STATEMENT OF THE PROBLEM

Planning for utilization of the behavior analysis process by a complex organization requires involvement by the whole health care team, including the patient, his or her family, and friends. Much of this involvement requires careful communication for the purpose of keeping the reinforcer under the control of the designated behavioral engineers: nurses, physicians, psychologists, therapists, family members, and the patient if he or she is directing his or her own program, as is the case in a self-control project.

Examples—teaching-hospital nursing unit involvement

One of the best ways to get involvement is simply to ask for it. Whom do you ask? In this example the clinical psychologist asked the nurse who would be most likely to be reinforced by a new idea for effective ward management–the head nurse. She accepted the description of the behavior analysis process as logical and agreed to invite the nursing staff to a series of three inservice meetings on the principles of behavior analysis to be presented by the psychologist. Her planning job was made easier because she had already established a weekly unit inservice meeting, to which the majority of the staff came every Monday from 2:30 to 3:30 PM. Her task was also made easier because she was supported by a nursing service department that believed that ongoing staff development was important and that allowed the participating evening nurses and night nurses compensatory time for coming in on their time off. The head nurse also had support from the assistant head nurses and the inservice committee, who accepted the invitation to include the series on behavior analysis within their inservice section on psychological adjustment; this section had been routinely presented to the staff three times each year. After the inservice series, the behavior analysis process seemed as logical to the staff as it had to the head nurse. The series had been particularly clear because the behavior of patients on the unit had been used as examples for discussion. The plan evolved into an agreement to start a pilot behavioral change case on the unit the following Monday. Graph paper would be used to document behavioral change; attention from the staff would be the patient's reinforcer; and the nurses felt that patient progress would be their reinforcer. Implementation of the plan is discussed in the following chapter.

It is prudent to give careful support to the head nurse and team so that their first experience can be a successful one. Relevant readings should be made available or should be easily procured. One rehabilitation unit requires its orientees to read a particular chapter on the subject during their first 2 weeks of employment (Krusen and others, 1971). Another unit makes a short article available to each new nurse; this article is short enough to be read on a coffee break (Fowler and others, 1969). Some units utilize an article on chronic pain (Fordyce, 1968). A pediatric unit distributes copies of an article on patient cooperation (Berni and others, 1971). Several rehabilitation units and several hospitals have available a nursing paper on nursing care audit and the problem-oriented patient record (Berni, 1971).

On some wards new nurses are given a one-to-one orientation to behavior modification techniques by the clinical nurse specialist. The nurse specialist in these instances is involved in most of the programs that call for the nurse to facilitate the patient's behavioral change; the specialist usually works closely with the clinical psychologist if one is on the case or on consult call. The orientees are supported by the nursing staff and the nurse specialist as they work with their first patients. During daily nursing team conferences there is an opportunity to discuss any questions about the behavioral management of patients. It is prudent to have resource people available for consultation as these behavior modification programs are going on. In most cases the clinical psychologist, the physician, the nurse specialist, and other members of the health care team are willing to discuss problems if they arise.

When the nurses have been selected by objective criteria, have access to some of the natural nursing milieu reinforcers, and have adequate information and practice, they usually enjoy their new role as behavioral strategists if they have set up a system of accomplishment identification, such as the system of problem-oriented patient records, with progress notes and accurate graphs or flow sheets. Their own success will reinforce continued analytical, systematic, and thorough problem-solving behavior. Successful behavior as a behavioral strategist will also be reinforced if it has been documented in routine, written evaluations leading to salary increments. Again, the problem-oriented patient record is a good source for the head nurse when the head nurse is writing the evaluation (this system is discussed in detail in Chapter 12). Staff picnics and snow-shoe trips help the new nurses feel the warmth of team solidarity; they learn to trust their peers, whose praise becomes reinforcing.

Example—teaching-hospital physician involvement

In this example, system planning followed much the same pattern as for the nurses with classes on the behavior analysis process that were presented by the clinical psychologist. Walking rounds were also utilized as teaching opportunities. Both the clinical psychologist and the head nurse attended medical rounds. The patients' physicians and psychologists attended nursing milieu meetings. The nurses identified the patients' behavioral problems, and the whole team brainstormed the problem solving together. Members of each discipline had an opportunity to learn from and to teach others informally.

Example—teaching-hospital allied health personnel involvement

The clinical psychologists presented continuing education seminars where each participant could plan a behavior modification program and share its progress with the group. Occupational therapists, physical therapists, and others had experiences in modifying a family member's behavior or their own behavior. This practice gave them experience in programming behavioral change and led to insight on how it felt to be a recipient of behavior modification—the patient's eye-view.

Example—teaching "private patient" health care team involvement

This example could occur in a large or small facility or in an inpatient or outpatient setting.

One team member—physician, nurse, social worker, or other discipline member—recognizes a behavioral problem for a particular patient and asks all the team members to meet at a special time to discuss it. The team member requesting the conference comes prepared to summarize the behavior analysis process and to outline and request a behavior modification program for the patient. If the team concurs, the initiating team member writes out the program and offers to present the principles and the program to any absent but participating staff, such as nurses on the night shift, or the initiating member arranges other orientation methods with the conference group. The patient and his or her family may also attend this first conference or at least a follow-up conference.

Example—patient-family self-control involvement

In this example the patient initiates the conference and plans his self-control behavior modification program. He may decide that he can afford a cassette for his tape recorder every 5 weeks if he has lost 5 additional pounds from his baseline. He may need to have his wife purchase the cassette at the appropriate time, and he may request the dietician to offer a particular diet. If he wants praise from the staff, it will be up to him to let them know his progress; otherwise the staff would remain neutral.

Example—nursing home or extended care facility involvement

The facility that is interested in establishing a prosthetic environment or an environment rich in reinforcers for patient progress toward self-care and independence may contract with a behavior modification expert to help them plan a facility-wide program. More than one discipline should be involved in the planning. One institution involved the administrator, nurses, social worker, therapists, one physician, several patients and family members, and community volunteer groups. Continuing education courses were planned for the staff, using the facility's own patients as participants.

Example—visiting nurse services, clinics, and private physician office involvement

The format for planning is similar to that in the previous example. The inclusion of several disciplines and community agencies is essential to provide the resources for effective reinforcers. The behavior analysis process is far from exotic. Many universities can now help interested individuals contact available experts. The bibliography at the end of this text includes several sources.

Example—teaching total hospital nursing service involvement

It is much more difficult to orient and support 300 nurses as behavioral engineers than it is to coordinate a smaller group of 30. However, more and more large nursing service departments are requesting assistance in planning the utilization of the behavior analysis process. One large hospital has asked experts to outline a workshop on the behavior analysis process for all the nursing personnel.

Although aides and practical nurses can be taught quite rapidly to perform behavior modification techniques, they need careful supervision and reinforcement by the professional nurse in order to maintain the continuity of the behavioral change programs.

System planning recognizes the importance of professional nursing staff selection when a hospital introduces major patient management programs, and fortunately directors of nursing are usually systematic in their selection. More and more the prospective employee's qualifications are evaluated against written criteria for a particular position classification, rather than by the old intuition method. These criteria are developed after the philosophy and the major goals of the organization have been established. As directors of nursing and administrators support management by democratic participation, the philosophy, goals, and personnel qualifications are updated by representative bodies of the whole organization. Continuing education programs within the department of nursing services help line staff to make better judgments as to performance qualifications and goals. Since their performance will be evaluated according to their contribution toward goal achievement, staff nurses are reinforced to take an active interest in goal setting. The concepts of consumerism and patient advocate help nurses to define performance goals. They ask themselves the question, "Did my action contribute to the patient's progress?" The question is a difficult one to answer, as you will see when we suggest in Chapter 12 a method of nurses' evaluating the results of patient care. The encouraging fact is that professional nurses want to participate in nursing care studies, and they want to participate in the planning and implementation of an audit method. They are interested in facilitating the solution or management of the patient's problems and are willing to be evaluated in this area as methods are refined. They are willing to attend continuing education classes on problem solving and behavior modification. Line staff nurses are interested in being evaluated on individual performance as well as team performance. They are also interested in being hired or fired by competent people who actually observe their performance. There are still occasions when the head nurse must ask a staff nurse to resign, but often is not the person who directly hires the staff nurse. As systems of accountability are developed, unit head nurses who are accountable for the results of staff performance will be reinforced to seek the authority of staff selection and staff retention or termination.

In this text we are looking at the selection of health team members best qualified to become effective in behavior modification techniques. Usually if they have demonstrated an interest in helping their patient solve problems and have demonstrated a willingness to look at both the patient's and their own behavior, they can learn effective behavioral change techniques.

Example—primary nursing involvement

As more nurse practice acts are updated and amended by increasing numbers of state legislatures, the role of the professional nurse is more clearly defined as including the direct responsibility and accountability to the consumer public for professional nursing practice. This responsibility and accountability to the patient is better met by the primary nurse who has direct 24-hour nursing responsibility for a specific group of patients until those patients are discharged or transferred into the care of another professional nurse. It is the primary nurse's responsibility to each selected patient to take a nursing history, to write an initial nursing care plan, to implement the nursing care plan, to implement certain segments of other disciplines' care plans, and to evaluate the quality, efficiency, and effectiveness of nursing care and patient response to that care, to modify nursing care as needed, and to write a nursing discharge or transfer summary.

In some locations, the primary nurse who fails the accountability responsibilities may cause the health care facility to be out of compliance and subject to decertification leading to closure of that facility. It is important for the primary nurse to insist on enough time to fulfill these responsibilities for the sake of personal integrity and professionalism and because of the increased threat of malpractice litigation due to the increased level of nursing salaries and the increased litigation consciousness of the public. In some large institutions, primary nurses are supervised by nursing coordinators and assisted by colleagues and other levels of nursing personnel. No matter how much coverage and assistance are effected, it still remains the responsibility of the primary nurse to maintain 24-hour excellence in nursing care for the assigned patients.

The primary nursing involvement gives more opportunity for a consistent behavior analysis process to be effected for patients when needed. It also is a behavior analysis system in its own right. As primary nurses analyze their behavioral responsibilities to their patients, they become more articulate to legislatures and the private sector regarding the need for basic reinforcers such as responsible compensation, sufficient numbers of competent and reliable nursing personnel, and sufficient numbers of competent and reliable expert consultants, particularly in long-term care facilities. They can describe that behavior modification concepts are useful in determining the importance of rewarding nursing home personnel amply and contingently if patients are to benefit from an enthusiastic and competent staff. They can point out that higher paying acute care facilities will then be less likely to drain off nursing home personnel, who have been carefully tutored on-the-job in the long-term care facility.

The primary nurse role provides opportunity for minimizing the old shift-to-shift nursing conflicts, because the primary nurse's nursing care plan will not be altered by another team member without direct communication with the primary nurse unless the patient's circumstance changes appreciably in a short period of time, such as the development of a fever. The primary nurses on the day shift brief selected nurses who will be caring for their assigned patients during the primary nurses' off duty hours and days off. The same communications among nursing shifts occur for the primary nurses usually scheduled on the evening and night tours of duty. These communications facilitate the behavior modification analysis systems planning because a carefully thought out plan has more chance for careful follow-through when it is not being modified every 8 hours.

Behavior modification analysis system planning can be effected in varied nursing care settings. The primary nurse in an intensive care unit can plan a reinforcement program for the patient to increase coughing and deep breathing with more probability of success if the patient, all other nursing personnel, the respiratory therapists, the physicians, and the family know and agree to the same plan, and if they all have assurance that someone, such as the primary nurse, is keeping everyone current on any modifications of the plan. Some orthopedic nursing units have welcomed a behavior modification program to help patients and assistive nursing personnel to remember to follow the procedures regarding the use of antiembolic stockings and therapeutic exercises consistently for patients who have had hip joint replacements. Often simple written tallies and honest peer and staff praise will be the only reinforcements necessary. When planning and evaluation are done consistently, the primary nurse is better able to know when to call or ask for a referral to a clinical psychologist for consultation. When the psychologist or physician initiates the behavior modification program, the primary nursing role gives nursing service a better opportunity to keep the health care team appraised of the patient's progress over each 24-hour period.

Example—certified nursing involvement

The American Nurses' Association divisions on practice have recognized competence as well as excellence in nursing practice under a broader program by providing two types of recognition for professional achievement; certification and diplomate status (*The American Nurse,* 1976). This is a new program, and it is certain to influence nursing service for some time in the future. Planning a behavior analysis system to be implemented by nurses and other health care professionals within a health care setting must include the knowledge of the changing competencies of these professionals. Since this is a book addressed to the nursing process, the nursing profession will be used as an example, but it is prudent for other health care professionals to identify the competencies of their members before planning behavior modification programs.

The American Nurses' Association's divisions on practice identifies *certification* to have distinctive eligibility requirements in specialized areas of practice, and identifies *diplomate status* in the American College of Nursing Practice to require certification and additional criteria for demonstrating excellence in practice. The Interdivisional Council on Certification requires the *certified* nurse to have: current licensure as a registered nurse; 2 years of practice as a registered nurse in a designated area of nursing practice immediately prior to application, 1 year of which may have been in an organized program of study in an institution of higher learning or in a continuing education program; and have current practice status in the American Nurses' Association's division in which certification is sought.

A *diplomate* has current American Nurses' Association certification in the designated area of nursing practice; is currently practicing in the area in which diplomate membership is sought; has 2 years of practice in the area of specialization post-master's; and has a master's degree in nursing or a related field from an accredited educational institution. Criteria and qualifications for excellence for continuing diplomate status are determined by the American Nurses' Association's divisions on nursing practice. These programs offer a variety of methods for state recognition beyond basic registered nurse licensure, and they may serve as a means of credentialing for the purpose of payment by third party payers.

Planning for cost accounting out the different elements of nursing practice will likely involve the identification of the level of certification of the practitioners and will probably help other health care disciplines plan behavior analysis systems with professional nurses because of a clearer understanding of competency. Similar changes in the clarification of competencies within other health care disciplines should, in turn, help nurses identify the consultants they might find most helpful in planning a patient's nursing care plan or behavior modification program. The essential elements in planning any system are effective communication, competency, and reinforcement of the planners. It is important that the planners find themselves compensated or reinforced in some way for their efforts, or good planning behaviors may become extinguished.

SUMMARY

System planning is the first step toward utilization of the behavior analysis process. The objective must be identified and orientation started before an effective system can be implemented. Many more experts are now available in behavior modification. Whether the project includes one patient or many, the principle of cooperation of all persons involved remains essential. Professional nurses have been prepared to participate in goal setting, problem solving, and accountability systems as they give health care. If they are included in the system planning, they are likely to be enthusiastic in the system implementation.

11
SYSTEM IMPLEMENTATION

STATEMENT OF THE PROBLEM

Implementation of the behavior analysis process requires reinforcers for patients, families, and the health care staff.

Example—teaching-hospital nursing unit reinforcement

Patient progress is perhaps the most potent reinforcer for the nurse, and a pilot case is a good way to ensure patient progress. For example, all the nurses knew the behavior modification program for a particular patient because they all had a part in its development. They monitored the patient's progress together and discussed their pleasure at change-of-shift report. This was a quadriplegic patient who needed to drink more water; it was a triumph on medical rounds to announce his major increase in water intake. The third opportunity for staff reinforcement was at their weekly milieu meeting.

Milieu meeting, or ward environment meeting, is so called because all the nurses from all shifts, the patients' physicians, and clinical psychologists are invited by nursing services to meet on the ward for the purpose of discussing patient problems and communication in general. Although this amounts to a total nursing time of from 12 to 20 hours a week, nursing services feels that it is valuable for nursing morale and patient care. A total of 7 hours of psychologist and physician time is likely to be donated to this hour-long meeting once a week. Nurses from different shifts and from their days off come in for this 2:30 to 3:30 PM unstructured discussion. Because many hours of valuable time are represented by the participants, the head nurse usually gets the meeting started promptly, and the nurses are ready to discuss the problems that may concern any or all of their patients. Medical problems as well as behavioral goals are reviewed, but usually at least one behavioral program is discussed or one is planned for implementation. Nurses have the opportunity to bring up what concerns them, but they also have time to share the ideas that seem helpful, giving each other positive feedback. A very important value is the opportunity to discuss patient problems and problem-solution planning with the psychologist and the physicians. After the behavior analysis process has been going on for some time, an equally important asset of milieu meeting is the opportunity for physicians and psychologists to give the nurses positive feedback regarding the outpatient care and the long-term follow-up reports on how the patients are generalizing their behavioral changes in their natural environment. On wards where inpatient gains can be very slow, this kind of feedback from other members of the health care team becomes a potent reinforcer.

Another planning and feedback system is the staff conference regarding one patient, sometimes called a panel session. Here the nurse and others working with this patient share information on patient progress and evaluation. The group during a panel session plan patient care goals and evaluate team and patient progress. At times the patient and his or her family are included. These sessions are helpful to the nurses' development only if they feel well prepared and participate constructively. The nurse who has relevant interactions with the team more than likely is positively reinforced to continue quality participation. By sharing the panel information with the nursing team, the nurse may have positive reinforcement for them. Peer reinforcement at daily team conferences and feedback reports from the visiting nurses about former patients add to the staff's progress.

Participation in recreation designed for and by the patients is a good way for the nurse to enjoy positive feedback from the patients and to observe the need for and to plan possible ways to help the patient generalize newly learned behaviors in the environment outside the hospital.

Last but not least, the informal coffee break, where one nurse teaches or reinforces another, gives an opportunity for frequent and fairly immediate positive reinforcement for the new nurse and veteran alike.

As research continues and new information is assembled, so should the nurse's education be on a continuum. Formal classes should be programmed for easy access on the ward. A revolving continuing education schedule is helpful to new nurses, and the review is useful to experienced nurses. It is important for the resource people to update their information in order to positively reinforce the experienced nurse's continued participation. Medical and behavioral subjects are usually included and presented by experts; in addition, the nurses prepare their own presentations from the literature and from their own experience. It is important that the schedule be flexible for the purpose of inserting special topics that concern particular patients on the ward; the inpatient example is obviously an advantage for facilitating learning because the nurses have an opportunity to practice the newly introduced behaviors during the patient's care. New feedback systems for the patients during behavior modification are examples that are discussed more fully in the chapter on future trends.

From time to time continuing education courses with behavior modification as an emphasis are available outside the hospital. The courses that incorporate an opportunity to rehearse the application of the information presented at the time of the course are apt to be the most useful. Most of these courses extend intermittently over a period of weeks.

An inexpensive but effective reinforcement for the nurse is to be asked to become a particular patient's one-to-one nurse. The nurse's name is placed next to the attending physician's name on the nursing care file as this patient's special nurse. Special expertise or rapport with this patient qualifies this nurse for this assignment. There will be other patients to care for, but the entire health care team will know this nurse is responsible for this patient's nursing care planning as long as he or she is in the hospital. The one-to-one nurse will write his or her nursing discharge summary and, if necessary, call in a public health nurse. Difficult patients usually do better with a one-to-one nurse, a result that is reinforcing to nurse, patient, family and team.

Solidarity is another potent reinforcement. This phenomenon of belonging, or being a member of a group, is reinforcing to many; it is also attainable by many. Again, how you manage this reinforcer is important. Are the group functions called just to discuss problems, or does the group gather to celebrate small and large successes? What behavior is necessary to be included by the group, complaints or accomplishments that make the whole group satisfied? How is a shy, productive nurse able to join the group, or how can the group function so that this nurse wants to join the group? How do you extinguish the behavior of a small, destructive group? All these questions can be looked at from a behavioral standpoint: what behaviors of solidarity reinforce productive work on the unit? These are the behaviors to reinforce. You may have to set up reinforcements for incompatible behaviors when nonproductive behavior is going on.

For some people money sounds like a coarse and mercenary reinforcer by which to motivate "angels of mercy," but nurses will attest that they also want a college education for their children and that money will buy it. The fact that money is a reinforcer is rarely disputed these days, but how it can be used or delivered receives much discussion. It is prudent for a person to be well aware of reinforcement schedules if he or she is responsible for using the organization's funds wisely. It is important to offer reinforcement for *results* and to document the results. It is aversive for one employee to see another employee reinforced for something he said he did rather than for what his actual behavior was. Who will take the time to work out appropriate and effective schedules for reinforcement? If the nursing administrator of the unit is responsible for the production of patient problem-solving behaviors and if reinforcement depends on that production, it is likely that he or she will take the time to reinforce the staff on an effective schedule. There will probably be a fund for special merit and the administrator write down the criteria for its achievement. Someone will say, "Yes, but what if your funds are limited, and you have two qualified people?" It is important that the nursing administrator set the requirements at a level that all must work to achieve; then the fund will be given on a first-come, first-served basis. A cycle of merit reward opportunities must be programmed to ensure that reinforcers will be available on a continuum. The most difficult problem is to identify the tasks, specific behaviors, processes, and results that need to be reinforced. A large group of system analysts, professional and amateur, from many disciplines including nursing are working on this very problem. Problem-oriented charting, which is discussed in Chapter 12, is one possible tool for the solution of this problem.

An advanced title, praise from respected persons, special conferences and trips, added authority and responsibility, special parking place (or, these days, any parking place), special dining room, private office—these items of status may be reinforcers to some individuals. Again, if you have only a few status symbols to award, you should be especially careful to watch the schedule by which you will assign them. Of course, the patients and families will award the nurses their most satisfying status symbol by expressing satisfaction in many verbal and nonverbal ways.

Patients and families are in the greatest need of reinforcers. From the day of the patient's admission you are in a position to learn from the patient and family what interests or pleases them. You can be alert to what the outside environment has to offer these people in the way of reinforcers. If swimming is important to your patient, you may be able to help him be an excellent swimmer through the re-habilitation center's recreational service. If the patient needs reinforcement from his spouse, you may be able to facilitate a private room for him to transfer to.

It is important to remember that it takes much patience to bring about change and much reinforcing encouragement both to staff and patients during early attempts with the process. Eventually their experience will be sufficient to the point that they will solve the most aggravating or worrisome problems.

Example—teaching-hospital physician reinforcement

Physician reinforcement can be described in two different ways, reinforcement for the physician and reinforcement by the physician. Patient progress and staff efficiency are usually two good reinforcers for the physician. His or her behavior can be modified toward more cooperation and communication with nursing staff if he or she knows that communication behavior yields consequences of patient progress and more efficient use of nursing time, which, we assume, yields more nursing time for more thorough care of their mutual patients. For example, the chain of events might start with a concise conference called by the nurse for the purpose of identifying for the physician the orders that appear to be outdated. The nurse might discuss with the doctor how time saved from the elimination of outdated orders can be used for the purpose of setting up an operant program to help one of their patients to drink more fluids. Carefully documented drinking-fluids behavior of the patient may show a major increase in only a few days. As a result of this patient progress, the physician should be well reinforced for communicating with the nurse.

Reinforcement by the physician can be extremely effective, because patients usually respect their physicians, or they would not have come to the physicians for care. The physicians' praise is reinforcing particularly if the patients feel that the praise is accurate. Nurses can help the doctors do a better job of reinforcing patients by seeing to it that the patients' progress records and graphs are kept up to date, complete, clear, and available. Reinforcement by physicians is important to another group, the nurses themselves. One way to reinforce a nurse to make an extra effort in the care of a difficult patient is for those interested in that care to listen to the problems the nurse identifies and to the plans suggested. The example can be expanded into a two-way street of the nurses reinforcing the physician and the physician reinforcing the nurses. Physicians may appear to be preoccupied with many serious decisions to make, but they know on what nursing units their patients receive the most thorough nursing care. They will listen as these nurses suggest behavioral change programs for solving some of the patients' problems. Even the busiest surgeon or internist will support the plans of competent nurses if their plans are concise, well documented, and defended by appropriate scientific rationale.

Example—teaching-hospital allied health personnel reinforcement

Nurses can help therapists reinforce their patients more realistically by keeping the therapists informed regarding patient behavior during the time the therapists are off duty. The nurses can help identify reinforcers and facilitate family communication with the therapists.

Example—"private patient" health care team reinforcement

Since the physician appreciates efficient use of time and since the spouse or relative often cannot afford to leave work, an evening conference scheduled during the physician's evening round may provide the answer to a conference time for everyone involved to discuss reinforcers. Many times the spouse or relative is the best resource for ideas of adequate reinforcers for the patient. If the patient has no close relative, a friend may be a good resource person to suggest reinforcers.

Example—patient-family self-control reinforcement

It is apparent that the broader and deeper life's interests are, the more reinforcers are available as one disciplines oneself toward self-control. Pediatric and school nurses are in an especially good position to encourage youngsters to develop many interests and talents. When the individual has learned many skills and has several different interests and satisfying activities, there are more reinforcers in his or her repertoire for self-control reinforcement. When the individual has varied interests, the family has more opportunity to help select reinforcers that might help the patient.

Example—nursing home or extended care facility reinforcement

Recently more and more interest has been generated in helping nursing home personnel find reinforcers for their geriatric patients.

For example, a rehabilitation center offered a behavior modification course to nursing home personnel. The objective read: to offer information and guidance to nursing home personnel for the purpose of modifying patient behavior during a patient problem-solving process. Requirements for the participating enrollees were twofold: (1) nurses are considered key persons in patient care, and (2) nurses bring to the first class a list of at least five of their patients' behaviors that they would like to increase or decrease. The class on principles of behavior modification was for 3 hours once a week for 4 consecutive weeks. After each class the enrollees went back to their home institutions and worked on the course project. Each week in class the nurses reported their progress. The instructor made a visit to each nursing home during the course at a time when the enrollee could discuss the behavioral change project. A final class 1 month later gave opportunity to evaluate whether or not the behavioral change described in the nurse's project lasted over any expanse of time. Had there been more funds, a second follow-up visit by the instructor could have been made 6 months later and would have better tested the question. It was interesting to note that all of the nurses completed their projects, had documented data, had a demonstration of behavioral change occur in their patients, and had developed a continuing education program for their staff (Sand and Berni, 1974). Two examples of projects were reversal of urinary incontinence and major decrease of inappropriate requests. In another instance, one of the nurses was able to find ways for a patient to bake cookies in an electric frying pan; this grandmother then had a real gift to give to her grandchildren instead of always having to be the idle recipient.

Example—visiting nurse services, clinics, and private physician office reinforcement

The important reinforcer is the natural environment, and knowledge of reinforcers in the patient's home and community is essential. Identification of reinforcers with which to help the patient maintain performance when he or she is at home can be achieved by the collective observations of visiting nurses and clinic staff who meet with the patient and family. Perhaps the visiting nurse is the one to pull this information together. However that may be, by sharing their observations, they help the patient and help themselves to achieve their objectives with the patient.

Example—total hospital nursing service reinforcement

The system by which nursing emphasis is guided by objectives and is evaluated by results develops reinforcers by its very nature. Participative management by the staff helps produce many natural reinforcers. When nurses see that their decisions and efforts help the patient, they are naturally reinforced to continue problem solving.

For example, many acute care hospitals are now interested in a program called "reality orientation" for the confused patient instead of waiting until the patient is discharged to a nursing home for "custodial care." Families are being introduced to this behavior modification program, which shapes in orientation to the patient's environment and orientation as to who he or she is as an individual. Attempts are made to teach calendar dates, what is going on in the news, and what is going on in the patient's neighborhood. Patients practice a busy daily routine, including exercises, cooking, project work, and perhaps a method by which a self-medication plan can be used without error. Staff may do some reminiscent therapy in conjunction with reality orientation, such as building an album of pictures of important occasions and of important people such as grandchildren. These memory books are well labeled so that the patient and staff can look at the book together and instantly know what the occasion is or who the person is. Time spent with staff looking at the memory book can be a potent reinforcer; it can also be a tool for shaping in reality and a "cue card" for daily reality orientation. Plastic picture cubes can be used in the same manner if they are carefully and simply labeled so they can be utilized by staff for frequent, short periods of time instead of gathering dust waiting for a longer period of time to be made available. Occupational therapists, psychologists, physical therapists, families, recreational therapists, and community resource people can help the nurse build a plan for a stimulating and reinforcing environment after discharge. It is certainly reinforcing to the nurse and other team members to see the individual return to home or a retirement home instead of having to be dependent upon a skilled care nursing home.

Behavior modification principles should be carefully used or the team effort will be futile, and the project will be punishing instead of reinforcing to the team and patient. It is interesting to note that many older people have to enter nursing homes because they have lost their housekeeping skills or perhaps they never really learned how to get housekeeping chores quickly and easily out of the way. An occupational therapist's skill in teaching an older stroke patient how to simplify his home management plus reinforcement for practice by the rest of the team made it possible for him to return to his own home. This example shows the importance of reinforcing independence behaviors before an individual is forced into a situation in which he or she rehearses dependency behaviors. As more accountability is established by patient outcomes, it may show increased cost-effective documentation of comprehensive rehabilitation and community services versus prolonged 24-hour skilled nursing home care. At present, home care is very expensive because much of the service is to people who have not had opportunity to learn independent behaviors in spite of disability. As behavior modification principles are more generally applied, the health care system may be advising adults to plan for retirement activities and living facilities which are reinforcing to independent behaviors; the old family home may become void of reinforcers and filled with barriers to independence and punishers of loneliness. If this is a possibility, adults should be advised to plan to choose a retirement living situation that is reinforcing and to choose it early enough for them to make new friends.

SUMMARY

Several factors are important in management of staff where behavioral change projects are being attempted: selection of staff against written, objective criteria; persons in leadership roles having actual authority and control over some of the staff's reinforcers; identification of possible reinforcers for staff; staff education, planning, and feedback systems; and an accountability system, which is mentioned again in the following chapter.

It is difficult to discuss implementation from any perspective without running into the words reinforcement or reinforcer. Since human behavior is the result of one kind of reinforcement or another, management of staff behavior should be relatively easy to systematize; the problem, of course, is that what reinforces one member of the staff may be aversive to another; or reinforcers may not be readily available. Fortunately, the same principles that apply to patient behavior also apply to staff behavior; perhaps an element of the environment can be programmed to become a reinforcer to one particular nurse.

In most situations behavior is not likely to change unless the immediate consequences to that behavior also change.

Perhaps the most important single factor for successful programs is that the whole team is reinforced for being consistent.

12
SYSTEM EVALUATION AND PROBLEM-ORIENTED CHARTING

STATEMENT OF THE PROBLEM

Evaluation of the behavior analysis process requires documentation of the patient's behavior change as to rate, quality, duration, and applicability to his or her problem.

ACCOMPLISHMENT AND PROBLEM-ORIENTED CHARTING

Nurses belong to a profession that still stresses individual human service and a job well done; otherwise young college graduate nurses would not stay long in a field where the salary is still comparatively low for the amount of responsibility and the number of unpleasant tasks involved. Nurses take particular interest in the individual patient, whose praise and progress are most reinforcing. Now nurses are learning that the patient's return to function is more important than this verbal praise if both are not available simultaneously. They are willing to hear from the visiting nurse that their patient is glad he was "made" to walk even though he agreed to but did not like the process at the time. Here is where a system of accomplishment identification is a useful reinforcer for the nurse who is asked by the patient to get him out of bed and get him going, but who at the same time complains about the difficulty he is having. We will share with you one system of accomplishment identification, the problem-oriented patient record; the original concept is outlined in Dr. Lawrence Weed's book on the subject (1970).

This system of identifying the problems of each individual patient on an indexed problem list in the front of his or her medical record is the key to the accomplishment identification on the part of the patient and each of the health care team members. The problem-oriented patient record includes patient identification, data base or history, and a dated, numbered, labeled, and systematically described list of patient problems. Any professional health care team member may add a problem to the problem list, but in so doing he or she must also add the same problem, dated, numbered, labeled, and systematically described to the patient's chronological progress notes. The team member's name and discipline must be indicated after each block of entries into the record, be it problem listing, problem description, or problem progress note addition (Dinsdale and others, 1970). The initial description of the problem should include: *s*ubjective data, *o*bjective data, *a*ssessment, and *p*lan for solution—SOAP.

For example, if Nurse Mary Jones initiates the patient problem list because she is the first person to see the patient, she is responsible for describing all the problems she lists. If, from her nursing history interview an examination, she had identified problem no. 5 as bowel incontinence, she will list and date the problem on the problem index list and describe it in the patient's progress record. She may write,

(Date)

#5 Bowel incontinence

Subjective data: Husband reports enemas given to patient about every 3 days. Last accident, yesterday. Patient used to go to the bathroom right after breakfast.

Objective data: Rectal sphincter tone present. Very soft stool on rectal glove examination. Rectum empty.

Assessment: Loss of normal bowel function caused by too many enemas.

Plan: (1) Evaluate bowel function for possible initiation of structured bowel program; start daily record on flow sheet.

(2) Omit enemas.

(3) Order bedside commode and commode cushion (Mary Jones, RN).

Since the hospital is using this medical record system, there are no nursing notes or physician progress notes; all disciplines, including physical therapy, and so on, are charting on the patient's progress record.

Mary Jones must be careful to be concise and to read the progress notes of all of the other health care team members in order to be up to date and to prevent redundancy. She initiated a flow sheet to be kept at the bedside for the purpose of keeping a daily, detailed bowel program record, which can be summarized in the patient's progress record once a week. Other examples of flow sheets are vital signs graphs, diabetic regimen summary sheets, continuously updated laboratory summary sheets, or an every 2-hour patient turning and positioning record sheet at the bedside. The turning record might have the initials of each nurse's aide as the task is completed, with room for comments. The registered nurse could summarize the aide's comments on the progress notes when appropriate; this way each health care team member's work can be identified, and the patient's progress or lack of progress can be documented regarding each problem. Mary Jones may later make the following notations on the progress notes:

(Date)

#5 Bowel incontinence

Objective data: See daily record on flow sheet.
Plan: Start structured bowel program (Mary Jones, RN).

(Date)

#5 Bowel incontinence

Objective data: See flow sheet summary included.
Assessment: Problem resolved (Mary Jones, RN).

Mary would then turn to the problem list index and check the "inactive" column opposite problem no. 5, giving the date and her initials. A nursing care auditor could identify each team member's contribution to the solution of problem no. 5 and could identify the patient's progress regarding that problem. Mary's peers, associates, employer, patient, and Mary herself could be reinforced by this accomplishment identification system. Each individual could identify success, usually a powerful reinforcer for most of us.

Patient problem identification and the problem-solving approach are not new concepts for nurses; but an all-team, patient progress record is new, and setting up the medical record as an indexed, scientific document can be threatening as well as reinforcing. If the health care team's successes are clear in this kind of document, so also are the mistakes. This fact, however, has not been an aversive stimulus for the professionals who have used this system consistently; rather, the systematic interdisciplinary record has been viewed as a useful learning tool, and again, most professionals are reinforced by their own learning accomplishment. Nurses have found that it is easier to practice this approach with their own nursing notes before transferring to the multidisciplinary patient's progress record (Bloom and others, 1971).

Several tools have been developed for the purpose of assisting in the process of nursing care audit; one tool has been designed to assist specifically with the problem-oriented patient record approach (Berni, 1972). As teams initiate the problem-oriented patient record system, they discover that it lends itself very well to the process of behavior modification. The use of the system produces a vehicle by which patient behavior can be identified, recorded, reinforced, and evaluated. For example, if the nurse is interested in increasing the patient's water-drinking behavior, the problem may be identified as dehydration. The subjective data may include the patient's statement that he does not like to drink water. The objective data may describe the dehydration physical signs and the quantitative behavioral data of just how much and at what rate the patient drinks water (baseline). The data may describe that attention from staff has reinforced other behaviors of the patient. The assessment may summarize the need for a behavior modification program. The plan may include a wall bar graph showing the patient's progress with his water-drinking behavior over each 24 hours. It may also include the team plan on how staff will reward his success with their attention when he meets his quota. The numbered, labeled progress notes offer a vehicle by which other team members can communicate about the plan's effectiveness or need for modification, such as comments from the physician or psychologist. After the problem has been resolved, it will be reinforcing for the whole team to see it checked off to the inactive classification on the indexed problem list.

One variation of the concept includes a column for physician's orders and a column for nurse's orders running down the right margin of the progress record pages. These orders are written at the time the plan is written. This procedure starts the implementation of the plan for the solution of the problem immediately. It also keeps the implementation record on the same document as the planning and progress record. The ward unit clerk could transfer the physician's and nurse's orders, such as medications and treatments, to the task nursing care file. The physician's medication order could go to pharmacy during the same process if the columns are backed by a second sheet of the no-carbon required, perforated paper. An example of doctor's order could be: medication X, two tablets every other day; the nurse's order could be, oral hygiene 6 times daily.

Several texts are helpful to the nurse working with the problem-solving process. One in particular has a useful problem identification appendix (Johnson and others, 1970). Another text describes implementation (Berni and Readey, 1974). This system can be used for patient problem-oriented team conferences, progress panels, care plans, discharge summaries, transfer summaries, and visiting nurse referrals. This system offers reinforcing feedback to staff, but also offers a nursing care audit accomplished by nurses rather than by accountants or some nonnurse systems engineer.

PSRO—PROFESSIONAL STANDARDS REVIEW ORGANIZATION

The passage of the Social Security Amendments of 1972, Public Law 92-603, 92nd Congress, H. R. 1, October 30, 1972, mandated the professional review of health care delivered to recipients of Medicare (Title 18), Medicaid (Title 19), and Maternal and Child Health Programs (Title 5). A part of this 1972 Act created the Professional Standards Review Organization (PSRO). The PSRO review is designed to assure that all health care is necessary, meets professional standards, and is provided economically in an appropriate health care setting. PSROs will begin by reviewing care in short-stay hospitals and in long-term care setting. This emphasis on quality assurance will give all of us interested in quality of life for the health care consumer an opportunity to document our plans for quality care, the application of that care, the consumer outcomes, and if necessary, the barriers to the application of quality care. This becomes a behavior analysis system, and the quality of the system will depend on the degree of alertness and on the behaviors of the health care workers.

The PSRO Program Manual describes the inclusion of the nonphysician health care practitioner in PSRO.

730. *Involvement of Non-Physician Health Care Practitioners in PSRO Review*

Health Care is provided by practitioners of a wide variety of health care diciplines. Review of care provided by non-physician health care practitioners should be performed by their peers. Thus, while the PSRO retains ultimate responsibility for decisions made under his aegis, it should seek the participation of all health care practitioners in the development of criteria and standards and the selection of norms for these professions, in the establishment of mechanisms to review the care provided by each type of practitioner and in the actual review of that care.*

---

*PSRO Program Manual, U.S. Department of Health, Education and Welfare, Office of Professional Standards Review, November 10, 1974. Chapter VII, p. 31.

Public Law 92-603
92nd Congress, H.R. 1
October 30, 1972

Social Security Amendments of 1972
Title XI—General Provisions and Professional Standards Review
Part B—Professional Standards Review
Declaration of Purpose

Sec. 1151. In order to promote the effective, efficient, and economical delivery of health care services of proper quality for which payment may be made (in whole or in part) under this Act and in recognition of the interests of patients, the public, practitioners, and providers in improved health care services, it is the purpose of this part to assure, through the application of suitable procedures of professional standards review, that the services for which payment may be made under the Social Security Act will conform to appropriate professional standards for the provision of health care and that payment for such services will be made—

(1) only when, and to the extent, medically necessary, as determined in the exercise of reasonable limits of professional discretion; and

(2) in the case of services provided by a hospital or other health care facility on an inpatient basis, only when and for such period as such services cannot, consistent with professionally recognized health care standards, effectively be provided on an outpatient basis or more economically in an inpatient health care facility of a different type as determined in the exercise of reasonable limits of professional discretion.*

It is important for health care professionals to take an active part in their local and national Professional Standards Review Organizations by assisting on local committees and by assisting their national associations as standards for patient care outcomes are established. The American Nurses' Association's publication, *Guidelines for Review of Nursing Care at the Local Level,* has been accepted by the National Professional Standards Review Council to be printed by the Bureau of Quality Assurance Health Services Administration as an official PSRO document. Expert nurses from many parts of the country were invited to Kansas City for the purpose of establishing criteria for standards of patient outcomes in response to nursing care. These nurses worked without compensation because they saw the importance of contributing to the standards which, in the future, are likely to be the same standards against which their behaviors and their patients' behaviors will be measured. The nurses identified criteria subsets, screening criteria, critical times, standard percentages, exceptions, and documentations in relation to target populations with

---

*"An Act to Amend the Social Security Act, and for other purposes," PL 92-603 92nd Congress, H.R. 1.

specified variables. They worked with the guidance of nurses who had attained the scholarly level of Ph.D. and who had experience in the identification and measurement of patients' responses or outcomes.

The American Nurses' Association's guidelines were tested in the field by other nurses and should have continued field testing and feedback in preparation for additional target populations assessment. The population titles chosen by the participants were:

1. Chronic illness—essential hypertension
2. Well population—family
3. Osteoarthritis
4. Nutritional deficiencies
5. Bedridden
6. Maintenance habilitation
7. Respiratory distress
8. First stage labor
9. Adolescent nutrition—Pregnancy
10. Management of the surgical patient—colostomy
11. Acute myocardial infarction
12. Management of the surgical patient—cholecystectomy
13. Depression, nonpsychotic
14. Alcoholism
15. Psychotic withdrawal

Sample sets of outcome criteria developed as part of the project were tabulated for the above populations (American Nurses' Association, 1976). This is difficult and often frustrating work but must be undertaken by the professionals involved if they do not want a behavior analysis system evaluation imposed upon them without their input.

The American Nurses' Association *Guidelines for Review of Nursing Care at the Local Level* will cost $3.00 when it is published. The Department of Health, Education and Welfare will distribute the publication to certain federal agencies in 1976.*

One way to evaluate the behavior analysis system is to take the concepts to varied facilities throughout a geographical region and attempt to see whether or not other health care professionals find the concepts useful in their settings and within the present limitations of their own settings, without adding additional staff. This was done in the state of Washington, and over 500 nursing home personnel were able to demonstrate positive behavioral changes in their patients

---

*Copies may be ordered from: The American Nurses' Association, Inc., 2420 Pershing Road, Kansas City, MO 64108.

130   *Behavior modification and the nursing process*

after supervised programs had been established. The behavior modification concepts were incorporated in a restorative nursing course coordinated by the Department of Rehabilitation Medicine, School of Medicine, University of Washington, Seattle, and directed by a rehabilitation nurse specialist.

The Department of Health, Education and Welfare utilized the curriculum, including all of the original behavior modification programs, for a model curriculum to be presented to the state health departments for use in restorative nursing courses. The problem-oriented medical record concept was utilized as an evaluation system for following the students' and the patients' progress.

In order to assist the reader to develop a visual image of the problem-oriented charting as a behavior analysis evaluation system, the following diagram is presented:

Problem-oriented medical record diagram*

Data base	+	Problem list	+	Initial plan	+	Progress notes
Patient assessment		Needs of patient		First plan to solve problem		Progress notes and flow sheets
What you know about patient		Symptoms and signs that call for change in patient's program or for more team effort		The start or beginning plan after interviewing the patient or family or others		Information after admission assessment
Patient's abilities and disabilities						*Progress notes:*
				Format:		Subjective Data—(described by the historian)
				1. Diagnosis, need for more information		Objective Data—(observed and measured)
				2. Treatment: Medication, Procedures, Programs		Assessment— (educated hunch)
				3. Patient, family, and staff education		Plan—(the same format as the *initial plan* format)
				4. Evaluation of the plan		*Flow sheets:*
				5. Goal or predicted patient outcome		(Continual records of many items)

*Adapted from Berni, R., and Readey, H.: Problem-oriented medical record implementation, St. Louis, 1974, The C. V. Mosby Co., p. 155.

PRACTICE PROBLEMS

There has been considerable space devoted to the presentation of system evaluation, including such systems as problem solving, degrees of certification, behavior analysis, quality assurance, and problem-oriented charting. All were presented within the context that the patient/consumer has a right to have competent care and to have competent assistance in solving his or her health care problems. We believe the nursing process is a logical and orderly way of doing nursing, and we also believe that any process usually involves the problem-solving system (Marriner, 1975). Perhaps with a patient care situation example, we can tie most of these systems together for the purpose of system evaluation.

The situation describes a 60-year-old male, Mr. Olson, who went into the hospital for prosthetic hip joint surgery, which was to replace a very painful arthritic hip. His surgery was successful, but he and his wife were anxious about the quality of nursing care. Several days after surgery, the nursing assistants inadvertently left his antiembolic stockings off for a period of 24 hours. He later developed thrombophlebitis, pain in the chest, and fever and was moved from the regular nursing unit to intermediate care for monitoring and more intensive anticoagulation therapy. The patient stated that he was anxious that the nursing personnel might forget to do something else that might be more important. He knew some doctors felt that antiembolic stockings were not absolutely necessary, but he was fitted with the stockings before surgery, and he learned later there was a written physician's order for continual antiembolic stockings, except for skin checks and bathing.

One problem for the nursing staff was how to prevent another patient's anxiety from developing under similar circumstances; how to prevent those circumstances from happening again. They looked to the following systems to help them:

1. The problem-solving system requires: collecting pertinent data; identifying the problem; planning a solution; putting the plan into action; and evaluating the plan.
2. The certification system requires: predetermining qualifications for competency of nursing practice; and predetermining the qualifications for continuing competency.
3. The behavior analysis system requires: identifying the behavior to change; monitoring the behavior to change; reinforcing the behavior to be increased; and withdrawing reinforcement from a behavior to be decreased.
4. The quality assurance system requires: setting standards for

patient outcomes in response to health care intervention; evaluating patient outcomes against the standards; and modifying discrepancies identified after the evaluation-audit.

5. The problem-oriented charting system requires: collecting a data base; identifying the patient's problems; writing initial plans for the attempt to solve each problem; and writing progress notes and flow sheets for the purpose of evaluating the care and modifying the care as necessary.

In team conference, the nurses conjointly remembered that the incidents of forgetting to put on antiembolic stockings for long periods of time had happened several times before, and since they had not solved the problem before, they called in the clinical nurse specialist, who was an assistant professor with the school of nursing. The group identified that the behavior to change was insufficient monitoring of patient care by the registered nurses. The base line was at least 12 incidents of different kinds of inaccurate nursing care interventions during the last month. The reinforcement was peer praise for those involved in changing the nursing behaviors and a ward party from the social fund if the incidents were no more than 1 during the first 2 weeks after the beginning of the program. The nurses realized that the nursing assistants needed more inservice and more praise for work well done, and they felt if they changed their own monitoring behavior, this would increase the probability of increased teaching and praising the nursing assistants at the bedside.

The nurses organized themselves as primary nurses with the help of their consulting nurse and began their program of more efficient nursing care monitoring and data collection 1 week after their team conference; this week gave the nurses time to get majority approval by their group and to establish guidelines for primary nursing as described in Chapter 10. The nurses were using problem-oriented charting already, but they modified their flow sheet headings to correspond to the patient problem numbers and titles. These flow sheets identified the nursing interventions for the nurse aides to perform on a task flow sheet and the interventions the professional nurses were to perform, including the items used for monitoring the aides and the items for patient teaching and for monitoring patient learning. For example, some of the items on the bedside flow sheet read:

Problem #2—Extremity circulation at risk
    a. Change the continuous antiembolic stockings q̄ 8 h. R.R.*
    b. Review exercises c̄ pt. q h (instructions at bedside). R.R.

---

*R.R. = Record Response.

For the same example, the registered nurses monitoring flow sheet read:

Problem #2—Extremity circulation at risk
   a. Check skin through stocking window q 4 h. R.R.
   b. Evaluate pt's exercises q 4 h. R.R.
   c. See total skin surface q d. R.R.

The nurses reviewed a handout on quality assurance and patient outcome and utilized a book to introduce themselves to patient care standards (Tucker, et al., 1975). The nursing consultant reviewed the primary nurses' plans, including the flow sheets and praised the nurses as they developed better systems for accurate recording of patient response to nursing interventions. The project succeeded, and no incidents of inaccurate nursing care were reported or observed in the 2-week period. The party was held and the nursing unit goal was set for fewer than 3 incidents each month with a party following if the goal was met. The consultant and the nursing coordinator continued to praise the primary nurses' progress and to record the same in the nurses' evaluation logs for their resumes. The nursing assistants also received reinforcers for their accurate nursing, including praise, attending the parties, and points toward salary increases.

If the project had failed, the nurses would have looked at the behaviors, the recording, and the reinforcers to see where the project needed to be modified. The nurses knew that tasks, monitoring, and teaching were not the only elements in the nursing process, but they felt that accurate nursing care was a good place to start. As they developed their standards of care and patient response, they felt they would be developing better quality of care as well as accuracy of care.

Self-test

Questions:	*Answers:*
1. List five steps in problem solving required to make a patient care plan.	1. Collect pertinent data; identify the problem clearly; write a plan to attempt to solve the problem; implement the plan; evaluate/modify the plan as necessary
2. Name the four major divisions of the problem-oriented charting system.	2. Data base; problem list; initial plan; progress notes and flow sheets
3. Name four divisions of the problem-oriented medical record progress note.	3. Subjective data; objective data; assessment; and plan
4. List five important points to review when writing an initial plan regarding a patient's problem.	4. Diagnosis; treatment; education; evaluation; and goal

5. What do the initials P.S.R.O. mean in the current health care audit system?

5. Professional Standards Review Organization

6. Name a 1976 publication by the American Nurses' Association on quality assurance.

6. *Guidelines for Review of Nursing Care at the Local Level*

7. Name three major elements in a behavior modification program.

7. Identify the behavior to change; monitor the progress of that behavior; reinforce the behavior to increase and withdraw reinforcement from the behavior to decrease

SUMMARY

We used to evaluate the nurse according to how many medical facts could be reiterated; how many tasks could be completed in an hour's time; how far the hair was above the collar; how good was the nursing care plan, which was done in pencil, erased often, and from which only the last notation was retrievable; and how the patient felt, with little attention as to where the patient had progressed because there was no written baseline to compare against where the patient has progressed from. With the use of systematic problem-oriented charting and care there is hope that all the health care professionals will document their complete data collection; their valid problem identification; their explicit and data-supported problem-solving plans of action and goal prediction; and their efficient plan application, modification, and ongoing evaluation. Weed (1970) suggests that the health care professional can rely on memory no longer; there is too much knowledge to remember. We suggest that the professional nurse continue to seek knowledge from the basic sciences, to sharpen problem-solving skills, to increase reading and data retrieval skills, and to be the honest, warm, meaningful person who is the patient's 24-hour-a-day advocate.

13
ETHICAL ISSUES

STATEMENT OF THE PROBLEM

Some of the treatment or patient management approaches described in this book represent a significant change from more traditional methods. As in any new approach, it is important to consider carefully whether or not there are abuses or misuses of ethical standards. We set forth in this chapter what we see to be the major ethical issues, and we make explicit how these behavioral methods relate to those ethical considerations. We also deal specifically with some of the more commonly encountered ethics-related questions that are raised by people new to the use of behavioral methods.

TREATMENT CONTRACT

When a patient enters some element of the health care system, such as a hospital, nursing home, extended care facility, or rehabilitation center, there is at least an implicit contract—and one that is, hopefully, as explicit as possible—as to what services are offered and what objectives are to be pursued. Since we are concerned here primarily with nursing personnel, we focus on that aspect of the health care team; but the points to be made apply to all health care professionals. As a member of the health care team, the nurse has an implied contract with each patient (and his or her family), as well as with the employing institution or organization. By agreeing to work within the organization, nurses also agree to do their best to further the health care objectives for each patient. That means agreeing to help the patient attain the objectives of treatment and avoiding doing things that may interfere with attainment of those objectives.

It is, of course, apparent that the specific objectives of a treatment program can vary greatly from patient to patient, just as they can vary from organization to organization and program to program. For some patients the objectives are to end the illness and restore full function. In other cases, such as problems of disability and many chronic diseases or conditions, the objectives are to maximize function in the presence of a disabling condition that will not itself end and that may even be a progressive condition tending to increase impairment. In yet other situations where the patient's disease is terminal, the objectives are concerned with optimizing the dignity and personal integrity of the person as he or she is dying. We cannot hope here to catalog all of the possibilities and deal with them separately. For the purposes of this book, we concern ourselves with situations meeting the following assumptions:

1. The patient or a responsible advocate (such as a family member or a member of the staff of a sponsoring agency) has requested professional help.
2. The effects of the professional help can be identified by decreased interference in the patient's life from the illness or condition or, in the case of progressive conditions, by optimal maintenance of levels of function consistent with the patient's medical condition.

Generally, those assumptions apply to nearly all hospitals, rehabilitation centers, nursing homes, extended care facilities, or homebound programs.

Setting treatment objectives

The first ethical point is that the patient or his or her advocate and the treatment or management program should agree on the objectives. Generally, most of those issues will have been settled explicitly or implicitly before the nurse has had much contact with the patient. That is, the general objectives should have been evident at the point of admission to the facility. This point concerns the nurse in several important ways. In the first place, as nurses begin to identify target behaviors, they are obligated to let those target behaviors be consistent and compatible with general program objectives. In the first chapter we cited the example of Mary, who needed to use the commode so that she could live independently. The target behavior of increasing use of the commode was exactly consistent with program objectives. In the second place, when the patient is uncooperative, it is important to assess whether the lack of cooperation means that the patient's efforts are taking him or her toward objectives incompatible with those implied in the treatment contract. We deal further with that point later in this chapter. For now, let us note that either health care professionals or patients may find themselves working toward objectives inconsistent with treatment goals. When uncooperativeness takes the patient away from treatment objectives, that needs to be made clear to the patient or advocate or both.

Respect for the individual

There is another implicit commitment in the treatment contract: to respect the patient as an individual. He or she is not a pawn to the professional's efforts, nor someone to be manipulated arbitrarily. He or she is not identical to any other patient. The nurse, as well as all other health care professionals, is ethically bound to honor this commitment.

Nurse acceptance of institutional goals

Another commitment here is important. When a nurse joins a program, there is implied acceptance of the general goals of that program. If the program has as its general objective to improve patient function and if a nurse is more concerned with helping the patient momentarily to feel better when to do so may delay progress toward the treatment objectives, that nurse needs to reassess to which set of goals a commitment has been made.

NURSE-PATIENT RELATIONSHIP

It should be evident from the examples cited in preceding chapters that a major element of these methods, as well as of other treatment approaches, is the nurse-patient relationship. It is sometimes the case that about the only effective reinforcer available to help a patient perform in the early stages of treatment is the positive value, regard, and attention of the nurse and other team members. If there has been little effort to establish rapport and to communicate effectively with the patient, one has every right to expect that treatment effectiveness will have been compromised. It is equally important to recognize that that treatment relationship influences patient performance. It can be used to help the patient, or it can be used in a way that will actually interfere with patient progress. That point, too, is dealt with in this chapter.

FREQUENT ETHICAL QUESTIONS RAISED ABOUT BEHAVIOR ANALYSIS METHODS
Is an incentive or reinforcement system a bribery system?

It is surprising how often the question, "Is an incentive or reinforcement system a bribery system?" is raised, when one considers that nearly everyone who raises the question is working for wages or some kind of monetary remuneration. Are wages bribery? We do not think so. If someone insists that wages are bribery, then we would have to say we are in favor of bribery. Wages and other programmed reinforcers are contingent upon work or effort. Incentive systems such as those described in this book are simply efforts to help arrange things so that those incentives, by becoming contingent upon effort put forth, help people to reach their goals. In contrast, bribery consists of incentives or reinforcers contingent upon crime or bad behavior, as when one tries to "buy off" the traffic patrolman who is writing a speeding ticket. Occasionally the argument is made that the nurse is bribing the patient by saying, for example, that the patient can earn visitor time by performing. If we assume that good ethical standards were followed in developing the program with the patient, then that promise of incentives being earned by performance is only an explicit statement of a contractual arrangement in which the patient is being encouraged to do the things he or she needs to do. The patient is not being encouraged to do things that he or she should not do.

Is withholding reinforcers a form of punishment? Do incentive systems punish patients?

If you withhold some of your attention from a patient who is engaging in a behavior that is to be decreased, are you punishing the patient? Similarly, as in the example of Lori in Chapter 3, if an amenity such as use of the radio in her room, previously available to a patient, is now withdrawn if she does not meet some performance contract, is that punishment? The answer is not simple. The answer depends mainly on whether the patient (or his or her advocate) has been a party to the formulation of the behavior change program. As noted in the chapter on punishment, in the strict technical sense any withholding of positive reinforcers can be defined as punishment. However, as we are using that term here, when a behavior change program has been worked out with a patient and in the course of that program there occurs a time when the reinforcers were not earned or when the behavior to be reduced has occurred (and previous reinforcers are being withheld), then rather than punishment, the patient has received another bit of help toward meeting treatment objectives. Moreover, consider what happens if the reinforcers are not withheld. Let us go back to the example of Mary in Chapter 1. Nurse attention was programmed to become contingent upon Mary's using the commode wtih Mary's knowledge and consent. If the commode was used, nurse attention was delivered; if the bedpan was used, nurse attention was withheld. If the nurses had not withheld attention when the bedpan was requested, they would have interfered with the patient's progress toward her treatment objectives by helping to maintain the interfering behavior: use of the bedpan. That is not punishment, but a thoughtful and ethical step toward important treatment objectives.

What about the case where nurses begin to withhold previously available reinforcers to a patient? Suppose, for example, that access to a TV set in the dayroom of a ward had been unlimited, but it was decided to let TV time be a reinforcer for a given patient. He or she might earn 30 minutes of TV-viewing time for each ADL performed in the morning. It is essential to gain the patient's agreement (or that of his or her advocate) to such an arrangement before going ahead. Once that is done, your program reinforces effective effort; it does not punish.

Are behavioral systems manipulative?

The charge that behavioral systems are manipulative of patients is perhaps the most common objection raised. We emphasize that such a charge may be true in any given use of these methods *or in any other treatment approach.* It is, of course, true that in one sense any kind of treatment intervention is manipulating the patient, for the professional is doing something that is supposed to have some influence on the patient. However, probably the key element in the question of manipulation is whether or not things are being done to the patient without his or her knowledge and consent. If you do something that influences the patient—whether it be behavior based or any other approach—and he or she does not know about it, you are manipulating the patient. If for whatever reason you carry out some behavior-based procedures without your patient knowing about it and if you have planned it well, you have every right to expect that his or her behavior will change; but you will have violated your ethical contract with your patient. Either the patient or, if your patient is for any reason incapable of weighing effectively the alternative consequences, his or her advocate should be involved in design of the treatment program.

Does patient awareness of a contingency management program interfere with the program?

Preceding statements about the importance of patient participation in design of a program indicate our view on the question of whether patient awareness interferes with the program. By all means, nurses should make their patients aware of the program. For that matter, so-called awareness does not make much difference one way or the other so far as program success is concerned. If, for example, you decide that you can help your patient most by paying little attention to him when he talks about his pain but being very ready to socialize at other times, we find that it makes little difference on effectiveness of your efforts whether or not you tell him ahead of time what you are going to do. That is, telling the patient that attention will be withheld when he dwells on his pain and will be given as freely as possible when he speaks of other things will not diminish the effectiveness of your efforts.

One problem that can arise about the matter of awareness occurs when a patient first learns that the nurses will withhold attention if he or she does whatever it is they wish him or her to quit doing. Some patients in that situation will receive more reinforcement from bedeviling their nurses by deliberately repeating the undesired behavior. Under those conditions, the impact of the withdrawal of nurse social reinforcers may be minimal. Of course, the nurse would have been both more ethical and wiser to have sat down with the patient and worked out a contract. Failure probably would have been avoided had the nurse elicited the patient's cooperation.

What do you do if your patient refuses to cooperate?

If your patient refuses to cooperate, you should first be sure there is agreement between staff and patient as to what the goals are. For example, the concern for the moment may be the performance of ADLs. Your patient is refusing to do them, and when you propose an incentive system, he says he is not interested and is quite content for his nurses to do those things for him (perhaps while promising he will do them faithfully once he is home). Your next step could be to go over with him why doing the ADLs is important to *his* goals. The chances are that will not be enough to get him going. Next you should pin down with him just how many ADLs are and are not being done each day. Once you and your patient are clear about that critical detail, the next step is to ask him what method he proposes to get more ADL performance. Notice here that the point of emphasis is that it is his responsibility, not yours, to get an ADL performance habit established. Your mission is to do what you can to help him accomplish that goal. At this point in the negotiating process, the patient is likely simply to promise to try harder to do better. Accept that as long as a record is kept of what he then does. Hopefully, he keeps the record, but you back up that observational method with periodic checks. If his promise to perform is not followed by an acceptable increase in performance, you are in a good position to go back to him and say something like, "Well, we tried it the way you proposed, and it does not seem to have worked well. These records show only such and such number of ADLs were done the past 2 days. Do you have another method you want to try to help yourself get going on this? The thing is that I have to do what I can to help you with this problem, and if the methods you and I use do not get us to the goal, I have to keep coming back to you. I am sure you do not want me nagging after you. You might consider an incentive system. Pick something you really want to do [be sure that what he picks is realistically available], and let that become your reward for performing." You can then go on to help him work out the details of such an approach. If then the reinforcer he chooses does not prove effective, as indicated by a failure of improvement in ADL performance, go back to him and help him find another incentive. Very often you can help a great deal by offering some special socializing by you or one of the staff; for example, someone will spend 15 minutes each evening chatting with him if he is able to accomplish his ADL quotas. The key point here is that it is so often unfortunately the case that these performance tasks end up seeming to be the responsibility of the staff rather than the patient. The result of the rebellious or relatively uncooperative patient is that the nurses nag him or her. The more they nag, the less performance they get because of course they are awarding to the patient special attention that he or she may not otherwise receive.

If the end product of your negotiating efforts with your patient is that you and he flatly disagree as to what the goals are, you are faced with a very different problem. If, for example, you see the goal as independence in self-care and the patient sees the goal as being in a treatment facility where people do things for him, the staff and the patient (or his family or advocate) need to get that problem straightened out. It is sometimes the case that these kinds of difficulties stem from misunderstanding by patient or family as to what the goals really are. When the patient or family or advocate, or both understand that the goals are such as you have expressed (assuming that you were correct) and they reject those goals, we do not know

on what ethical or logical basis a program could continue to work with
the patient.

Do behavioral methods interfere with personal freedom?

The concept of personal freedom is not simple. The concept does
not, for example, mean that a person has a license to do anything
he or she chooses to do. There are always legal, practical, ethical,
and social constraints on our behavior and our choices. Personal
freedom can be thought of as the right to have as many free choices
of action as are consistent with the restraints imposed by the rights
of others in the situation in which the person is involved.

As the issues of personal freedom relate to being a patient or client
of health care services, we think we have shown in this book that
behavioral methods give patients more awareness of and participation
in goal definition and the manner of working toward those goals than
is often true of other approaches. To the extent that we are correct
in this statement, the patient has as many or more choices of action
in behavioral systems. As noted above, for example, when we discussed negotiating new contracts with an uncooperative patient, the
patient has many choices as to goal identification and methods for
getting there. Above all else, when these behavioral systems are being used in an ethical and practical way, the patient always has the
choice of earning or not earning the reinforcer.

In this context, one could ask whether a patient has the right to
decide not to perform tasks deemed essential to his or her care. For
example, does a patient have the right to refuse to perform ADLs if
those tasks are judged to be essential? The answer depends on the
nature of the treatment contract. To illustrate by taking an extreme
but not uncommon situation, let us consider an elderly patient who is
without family and is supported by public assistance funds and who
is admitted to a nursing home essentially for maintenance objectives.
That is, it is anticipated that he will not regain sufficient function to
permit him to live outside an institutional setting. Let us further suppose that this patient has preserved enough of his mental faculties to
be able to understand reasonably well what is going on around him.
The staff of the nursing home have an obligation to the patient to
give him the best care they can. They also have an obligation to
the sponsoring agency, in this case welfare or public assistance and
its supervisory mechanisms, to provide acceptable standards of care
to that patient *and all other patients* sponsored by that agency in that
facility. In addition, of course, the staff of the nursing home have an
obligation to provide acceptable levels of care to all other patients in

the facility, regardless of who sponsors them. Now let us narrow down our example to the single question of whether the nursing staff have the right to take steps to increase the chances that the patient will feed himself (assuming that he is physically capable of doing so) when he decided he prefers to have a nurse feed him.

If nurse time spent feeding the one patient significantly interferes with the nursing staff's ability to meet their other obligations, those nurses are obligated to try to help this patient take over the feeding process. Stated another way, personal freedom for a patient does not include the right to deprive other patients of needed nursing care and attention.

The steps those nurses might follow in working with the patient to help him take over self-feeding might well follow what we stated above in discussing the uncooperative patient. In this particular case, it would be important to explain to both the patient and the appropriate representative of the sponsoring agency what steps are contemplated and why.

The kind of example cited was deliberately chosen to represent one of the more difficult kinds of personal freedom issues. The principles that we have followed here will be reasonable guidelines in most problems of this sort in the nursing context.

Who is qualified to use behavior modification methods?

The question of who is and who is not qualified to use behavior change technology in human service settings needs to be considered. This issue can have legal, ethical, and territoriality implications. We have no more competence or information about the specific legal issues which may be involved than does the reader, for legal constraints depend upon the particular setting (e.g., hospital, nursing home, visiting nurse program) and the legal jurisdiction (e.g., which state, which county, which set of institutional rules). We shall, therefore, forego discussion of the legal issue except to note that behaviorally based treatment interventions must meet the same legal criteria as other human service interventions.

The ethical concern, in the more limited sense of who is or is not qualified to use these methods, clearly is rooted in the ethical constraint to which all health care or human service professionals are committed; namely, not to hold oneself out as competent to do or to undertake to do methods or procedures for which one is untrained. That statement leaves unresolved in the specific instance the definition of "sufficient training." How does one know whether he or she is sufficiently trained?

Application of the methods and procedures described in this book may be divided into two parts. The first, and by far the most complex, is to decide or determine what behaviors should and/or can be changed. That is the task of behavior analysis. It is a kind of diagnostic task. Some health care workers are insufficiently trained to undertake entirely independent diagnostic or evaluation programs in health care settings. However, once safe and prudent parameters of behavior are identified by the diagnostic process (Can this post-myocardial infarction patient walk X amount? Does the right brain cerebral insult in this stroke patient permit safe independent ambulation?), there remains the second and equally important mission of doing something about the problem.

The methods described in this book represent a technology by which one seeks to attain goals defined broadly and limited by the diagnostic process. The mission of this book is to help health care professionals to use this technology to those ends. The amount of training readily realizeable from this book is not likely to suffice to analyze or evaluate complex patient problems during the diagnostic phase of patient contact. The methods should prove sufficient to permit one to proceed with the behavior change process once diagnosis has outlined prudent limits. Having stated that in a general sense, it should be added that people are complex. Their behavior patterns represent a complex interplay of many forces, both extant in their current environments and as represented in their repertoires by prior experience or learning. It follows that simple changes in contingency or reinforcement arrangements to a bit of behavior is by no means automatically ensured of success in changing that behavior. Experience indicates, however, the methods described in this book indeed have considerable potential for helping people to make important behavior changes. The methods are no panacea and no "sure thing." But they *are* effective, and the cost of their use in time and effort is usually very rewarding.

We can now come to the territoriality issue. Behavior change methods do not belong to behavioral scientists (in the formal use of that term) or to clinical psychologists or psychiatrists, and the like, anymore than pupils belong to teachers, children to pediatricians, or patients to nurses. The methods speak for themselves. They are for use in human service settings. The user needs to know when and how to use them. The user needs to have enough wisdom, integrity, and self-confidence to know and recognize when something is going wrong and to seek additional consultation. When a behavior change effort seems to be getting into trouble or is not advancing, additional advice or guidance from someone more experienced in the methods should be sought.

In the practical case, our judgment and experience lead us to suggest that, as a general rule, it is wise and helpful to initiate behavior change methods in a health care setting with a back-up system of consultation from someone with experience in the methods. That consultant is likely to need to play a steadily diminishing role as experience develops.

14
FUTURE TRENDS

The professional literature for the helping professions shows a rapid increase in the past few years in the kinds of settings in which behavioral methods are being successfully applied. In this chapter we deal with some of the more important trends that we think will be worth your while to follow. We also call your attention to other readings that will be helpful supplements to what has been presented here.

The underlying theme of this book is that it is useful to look at patient care in learning or behavioral terms, although we do not mean to suggest that you should use only behavioral methods. We anticipate that time and experience will reveal even more applications of learning methods in health care systems. A few examples of possible applications follow, and in some instances we cite literature references to illustrate what can happen.

CHRONICITY AND LEARNING OPPORTUNITIES

Behavioral methods have many applications in acute as well as chronic care situations. In the matter of care of the chronically ill patient, however, these methods and concepts take on an extra importance. One of the major implications of viewing the chronic care process in learning or behavioral terms is recognition that chronicity means repeated opportunity to learn. The patient with the problem and those working with him or her are likely to develop systematic ways of behaving in relation to the problem. The patient will do certain things, such as ask for help, do things for himself, complain, or withdraw. The reactions of the nurses, family members, and nearby patients may be seen as potential reinforcers. The key issue is whether those reinforcers are attached to effective or ineffective behavior.

NURSE REINFORCEMENT OF ILLNESS BEHAVIOR

A nursing staff, by their behavior, can support effective patient performance. They can also respond in ways that support or teach poor performance. Family members and other patients have the same potential. We have made this point before. In Chapter 2 when we noted that nurse attention, when it becomes contingent upon something going wrong, as in limiting nurse interaction with a patient to nagging him or her to do something, can easily serve to reinforce and thereby strengthen the very behaviors that should be reduced. We make the point here again because, in our view, the extent to which many routine methods used in management of chronically ill patients have a tendency to reinforce undesired responses is only beginning to be appreciated. As the truth of this point becomes more apparent, we can anticipate that organizational procedures in chronic care facilities will begin to undergo further change.

A number of years ago Ayllon and Michael (1959), working with a group of psychiatric nurses in a mental hospital, were, simply by reprogramming nurse responses, able to help a large number of patients previously dependent on the nurses' help in eating to begin to feed themselves quite effectively. They had discovered that the nurses were systematically responding in such a way as to encourage need for assistance rather than independence in feeding.

In this book we have provided a number of illustrations of how nurse response to individual patient behaviors can influence what the patient does. This kind of analysis of patient-staff interaction needs to be made about many nursing routines. We expect that many chronic care routines will be found to promote dependence or less effective patient performance. Another example to illustrate this point is work by Fordyce and his colleagues (1968, 1973, 1976). They have shown that conventional methods for handling pain medications in problems of chronic pain may have the effect of promoting rather than inhibiting addiction or habituation. When pain medications are put on a prn, or "take only when needed," basis, the result is that the patient's expressions of pain are systematically reinforced by receiving medications, and absence of pain is never reinforced by medications.

If the medications in fact have potency in reducing discomfort, certainly a likely event, than one has every reason to expect that they can serve as reinforcers to strengthen such pain behaviors as visible and audible signals of pain and asking for medications. In behavioral terms, pain medications, given on a prn basis, become pain contingent. Changing that arrangement so that medications become time contingent rather than pain contingent can help reduce both addiction or habituation and, in some instances, the pain itself. Their procedures should be studied in more retail before one attempts to apply them. Details of the procedure are in Fordyce (1976).

Once we recognize that a nursing or chronic care unit is fertile soil for learning because of the extended intervals in which there is opportunity for systematic relationship between patient behavior and staff response, the search for ways in which we are reinforcing the wrong responses can become both intriguing and helpful. We expect that this kind of self-inspection will continue and will reveal more ways in which nursing methods actually make nursing jobs more difficult and impede rather than assist patient progress.

SKILL LEARNING

What the chronically ill or disabled patient needs to begin to do once he or she enters that state of chronic illness can be thought of as a set of skills. This points to yet another way in which learning concepts are pertinent. In Chapter 7, we called attention to the importance of breaking a skill or task into simple components and then systematically reinforcing each component as it is mastered and added to the repertoire. This book has tended to focus on patient care problems. The techniques described, however, are equally pertinent to learning a skill. To what extent, for example, is the process of teaching a patient colostomy care or catheter irrigation organized in such a way as to use reinforcement principles to their maximum effectiveness in helping the patient learn? To what extent is the process of helping a recently disfigured patient, or one who has recently become confined to a wheelchair and feels quite self-conscious about being seen in that state, to quit withdrawing and begin to interact with others programmed in such a way as to let reinforcement principles go to work to help him or her over what are for the patient very tough hurdles? Is coaxing, encouragement ahead of time to try, or exhortation the approach? Sometimes that is enough. Often it is not. Why not put nurse socializing to work in a systematic way by accompanying the patient in those first ventures out of social isolation in his or her room and toward other patients or public areas of the hospital or nursing facility? The nurse then is systematically reinforcing successive approximations toward independent socializing.

AUDIOVISUAL AIDS

Shaping and programmed learning principles have been playing increasing roles in the educational process. These same methods are becoming more available as aids to nurses and other health care professionals. There are, for example, an increasing number of closed-loop, single topic films that can be used to teach patients and family members, as well as nursing personnel, a number of skills in such things as doing transfers from bed to wheelchair or wheelchair to tub, in dressing when one hand or arm is nonfunctional, as in stroke patients, and so on. It is very useful to utilize very short films that break down a skill into its component parts. The approach follows good shaping principles. The nurse or therapist can supplement the film with an organized reinforcement program whereby each increment in performance is reinforced by any of a variety of methods. The nurse may, for example, provide social recognition in the form of a graph at the patient's bedside that portrays progress, as well as give direct approval for the patient's efforts. We can anticipate that more and more effort will be made to program or package the learning process for specific patient (and nurse) performance skills through the medium of video tapes, closed-loop films, and so on. Those methods will often prove helpful. When they are supplemented by use of reinforcement methods by the skilled health care professional, their impact will become even greater. An example of an effective patient self-teaching package is "Wheelchair Accessability—Opening the Door to Housing."*

FAMILY INVOLVEMENT

At a number of points in this book we have made reference to the role of the family in patient care. In Chapter 13 on ethics, for example, we noted the importance of involving the family in definition of treatment goals. We also noted how they can help to find and deliver reinforcers. In our view, the family is underutilized as a treatment resource. One result is that some problems arise that need not arise. Because they are not involved enough in the process, family members may not understand and appreciate all of the treatment or management goals and methods. They also may be reinforcing the

---

*By M. Wittmeyer and J. Barrett, Health Sciences Learning Research Center, University of Washington, Seattle, 1976 (28 minutes).

wrong responses, thereby working at cross-purposes to the treatment staff. Finally, it is usually the case that they want to help but do not know how. A little time spent informing and instructing family members on how to systematically reinforce some patient behaviors and on how to withdraw reinforcement from others can go a long way toward helping with patient progress.

Examples such as those of Bushell and Jacobsen (1968), Wahler (1969), Zeilberger, Sampen, and Sloane (1968), Patterson (1971), and Shelton and Ackerman (1974) illustrate further ways in which family members have been put to work in helping carry out contingency management programs with clients or patients. Reference was made earlier in this chapter to work by Fordyce and his colleagues with selected problems of chronic pain, using reinforcement principles. It can be added here that ordinarily a patient will not be admitted into that program unless the family agrees to participate systematically in the use of reinforcement principles in the treatment program. Other illustrations of this basic point are found in numerous projects around the country in which mothers are being pressed into service as teacher aides in Headstart reading programs with disadvantaged preschool children. There is every reason to expect and encourage increased training of family members as adjunctive therapists. More particularly, one should expect increasing efforts at training family members in how to support effective patient performance through selective reinforcement—both in the hospital or nursing facility and at home. This book should prove a useful reference for family members to prepare themselves in the use of reinforcement systems. Other useful source books or training manuals for family members are the works by Patterson and Gullion (1968) and Patterson (1971).

In this chapter so far we have limited our concern to training and maintenance of performance of patients and family members. We shall now consider some questions and future trends with regard to staff performance.

NURSE REINFORCEMENT

Baer and Wolf (1967) in their excellent article on generalization make the comment that behavior, like the flower, does not automatically bloom. Behavior will occur if it is reinforced and will diminish and eventually stop altogether if it is not reinforced. That is no less true of health care professionals than of patients and their families. In the Preface to this book and in Chapters 10, 11, and 12 we raised a number of issues regarding the importance of applying reinforcement principles to staff as well as patient behavior. We noted, for example, that helping nurses to change their methods will require more than simply informing them about new methods. It will almost certainly be necessary to provide special encouragement and reinforcement during the early stages of utilization of any new methods until results become apparent enough and strong enough to maintain their efforts. We have also called attention to how some routine procedures in patient care may actually be working against, not for, patient progress—though we are by no means suggesting that was the intent. Let us take this point a step further. It seems to us that some chronic care programs are organized in such a way as to make it difficult for staff to take additional action to provide more help for more patient progress. A hypothetical example will help illustrate the point. Imagine a nursing home with a 50-bed ward of primarily elderly patients who have limited mobility, but with help in getting started, are capable of independent ambulation. Let us suppose that a minimum of three walking trips a day the length of the ward corridor, perhaps to a dayroom or dining room, would have several beneficial effects. It would help minimize joint contractures, improve circulation, provide mental stimulation, and slow down withdrawal into ruminative fantasy. It would also increase the chances that patients would have to interact with each other, thereby helping to make each patient a potential contributor to the welfare of fellow patients.

What about the line staff on that ward? What are their reinforcers? Which of their behaviors are being reinforced? In some instances, for example on an evening shift, the work load may be considerably lighter if staff members do not take effective action to get their patients out of bed and walking about the ward. If they do try to get them up (when such has not been the routine in the past), they will likely have to provide physical assistance to some patients in getting them to their feet. To avoid falling, some patients may require standby assistance while walking. Some patients will, particularly in the early stages of such a mobilization program, be quite reluctant and openly resistant. Anyone familiar with nursing homes will know that simple reasoning with the patients is not always the answer. Here we have a situation in which ward personnel are asked to perform what may be a fairly arduous and difficult task. What are *their* reinforcers? If the organization of that ward relies on signs of patient progress as the major and virtually sole source of reinforcement for such efforts, the ward is going to find itself in trouble. In the first place, not all people working in health care facilities are reinforced by signs of patient progress—though, fortunately, most of them are.

In the second place, those signs of patient progress may be quite remote and even hard to see. The withdrawn patient who is induced to walk around the ward does not stop being withdrawn. He or she may begin to show less withdrawn behavior. Knowing that the proportion of patients on a ward who have severe joint contractures has gone down by 35% is not a certain way to reinforce all ward personnel. Even if it were, that kind of reinforcement does not begin to occur for quite some time after starting a mobilization program. As has been noted earlier in this book, reinforcers, if they are to have influence on behavior, need to be delivered promptly—particularly in the early stages of a behavior change process.

Consider what may happen to our hypothetical evening shift personnel if they do not help get the patients out of bed and walking. If the nursing hierarchy on that ward is not providing adequate inducement for them to perform, these personnel are likely to find that their shift of duty is lighter rather than heavier if they do not work at getting their patients out of bed. What are the charge nurse's reinforcers? She undoubtedly will be influenced to some degree by signs of patient progress, but we make her load very heavy if we rely solely on that source of reinforcement. If she behaves less militantly about getting her staff going to mobilize the patients, she will be to some extent reinforced by fewer complaints about work loads. It is even the case in some nursing home facilities that the financial inducement to the institution for patient care increases if the patient is defined as bed bound. That arrangement can have the effect of providing some monetary reinforcement to the administration for not making special efforts to mobilize patients. This kind of hypothetical situation of course exists to some extent in reality. We do not know how much or how often. We are sure that it occurs more than any of us want. Our major point in raising this issue here is that it should be recognized that institutions may function in such a way as to reinforce behaviors that work against optimal patient goals. In such a situation, nurses working there need to explore alternative ways of providing reinforcement for their line staff. A number of possibilities exist. Special incentive systems that are aimed specifically at patient mobilization can be set up. The incentives used could be very modest cash rewards to ward teams showing the greatest increment in patient mobilization, or an occasional extra day off for "winning" performance. It may often prove sufficient to post performance records so that individual staff members can gain recognition for having effectively promoted increased walking in a group of patients with whom they have been concerned.

INSTITUTIONAL REINFORCEMENT

Reprogramming of incentives within health care facilities in order to let those incentives be aimed more precisely at patient welfare rather than, for example, staff convenience, is likely to become increasingly common. There are indications too numerous to mention that our health care system is undergoing increasing scrutiny from the perspective of accountability of performance measurement. Insurance companies, for example, are not so much interested in how many patients you treated as in how many of your patients became independent in self-care or stayed out of the hospital or returned to work. More and more of the proposed public insurance programs are moving in the direction of letting fees to health care facilities be governed by service achievements, not units of service rendered. Stated another way, the performance of a program increasingly is coming to be evaluated by what patients do—that is, by changes in what they are able to do—not by whether or not they received services. Chronic care facilities will need to be able to arrange their programs so that staff performance is aimed as pointedly as possible at optimal patient performance. The processes of behavioral analysis and problem-oriented charting are exactly pertinent to these trends. We wish to suggest that as your patient care programs develop increasing mastery of behavior analysis systems, including problem-oriented charting, you will thereby have taken an important first step toward being able to identify with some precision the effects of your programs on your patients.

PROSTHETIC ENVIRONMENT

Let us consider briefly yet another trend that seems likely to play an increasing role in management of the chronically ill patient. Parallel advances in bioengineering and behavioral science and the pairing of these two fields have led to some very interesting and productive developments. We are concerned here with two such trends, what Lindsley (1964) has called the prosthetic environment and biofeedback systems.

The concept of the prosthetic environment refers to more or less permanent changes in the physical or functional characteristics of the environment in order to enhance and sustain patient performance. It is contrasted with the therapeutic environment, in which there is a temporary situation (treatment) designed to change how much a person can do, with the expectation that he or she will go on to use the new repertoire after treatment is completed. For example, teaching a patient how to maintain sitting balance and how to rise safely from

reclining to sitting and from sitting to standing is a task of a therapeutic environment. After being taught how to do this, presumably
the patient would then continue to do it. Putting side rails on a bed
to keep a patient from falling to the floor, if it is a more or less
permanent arrangement, as is necessary for some brain-damaged or
senile patients, illustrates the prosthetic environment.

We need not concern ourselves with details about the concept of
prosthetic versus therapeutic environment. The major trend to be
noted is the increased use of various devices designed to promote
either patient performance or patient learning. The work of Halpern
and Kottke (1968) is an example. We shall cite several individual
case examples from our own experience to illustrate further the
kinds of approaches to which we refer.

One elderly lady with parkinsonism was noted frequently to lose
her balance in her wheelchair and to fall to the left so far that she
could not regain her balance. She would have fallen to the floor were
she not restrained by a belt. The problem was to get her to detect

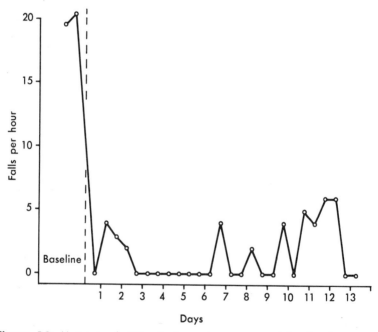

Figure 10. Maintained sitting balance by automated feedback (tone) in
a brain-damaged patient (two 30-minute observation or training sessions).
Patient entered a rapidly progressing terminal illness approximately on
day 10; project was soon ended.

falling soon enough in the process so that she could stop herself from going beyond the recovery point. She fell over every few minutes, so often that it interfered with whatever activity she was engaged in, to say nothing of the frequent necessity for staff members to stop what they were doing to come restore her to an upright sitting position. The solution was to position an electric eye on the back of her wheelchair in such a way that when her head and shoulder moved a very few inches to the left in the early stages of a fall, a tone sounded. Figure 10 shows the results of this procedure. She was observed for an hour first, during which she fell 20 times, or approximately once each 3 minutes. As Figure 10 shows, all she needed was to hear the tone a few times, and then she was able to detect the early stages of a fall and thereby prevent it from happening. Conceptually, the process was to redesign her environment so that whenever a certain event occurred (leaning 3 inches to the left in her wheelchair), a signal sounded.

A patient in his mid-50's became almost totally paralyzed from the neck down because of a neurological condition. He would awaken frequently at night and, being unable to move his arms or legs or body, often would become frightened that no one was around to help him should there be congestion in his throat for which he had only limited ability to cough. His nurse call switch was positioned so that he could call his nurse by turning his head to exert pressure on a cheek switch. He would do that frequently, but he would also call out in an incessant yelling because by that method he could gain quick reassurance that someone was indeed close by to help him if he needed it. In a matter of days the nursing staff was being run ragged by as many as 200 calls in a night. The patient was destined to return home to be cared for by his wife. Obviously, if he continued the night calling with any frequency, his wife would lose her sleep and soon become incapable of caring for him. It was therefore essential to reduce the frequency of night calls, without prohibiting him from calling when it was essential for him to do so. The remedy followed was to set up a counting device that displayed the count in inch-high luminous digits, which were clearly visible in the dark. The counter was positioned in his room where he could see it. Nurses could advance the count by pressing a switch. They did so each time he called out, though they also answered his calls. All of this was explained to the patient at the outset. After the baseline, or typical rate of calls per night, was counted, his nurses negotiated with him a quota of calls for each night. He was very quickly able to bring the number of calls down sharply. Conceptually, what had been done was to provide him with continuous information as to how much he was calling. When he could see the current count in the dark, he knew his needs were being met.

The number and kinds of devices that might prove useful is limited primarily only by our lack of imagination. Consider further the situation discussed previously, in which we were concerned with mobilizing nursing home patients. It would not be difficult to make a device that would record a number and sound a tone each time the patient took a step. Both the count and the tone could be reinforcers. The device would probably be needed with only some patients and then only during the early stages of a mobilization program. After walking had progressed to where the movement cycle could become a trip around the ward, the device could then be used by another patient. For those patients for whom the count or tone were reinforcers themselves, or where the count won tokens that could then be applied to other reinforcers, the device could save any number of nurse manhours while providing more accurate and systematic reinforcement for patient performance than the busy nurse could ever hope to deliver. Our point here is that nurses should look for and expect various automated reinforcing and feedback systems to emerge that will enhance nurse effectiveness by permitting more intensive and more consistent reinforcement for even small units of behavior.

BIOFEEDBACK

In recent years the process of biofeedback has emerged as a significant new treatment approach to a variety of patient problems. Biofeedback consists essentially of arranging that the patient will receive immediate and very precise information about the current state of some body part or process. For example, a patient may be fitted to a device that will measure his blood pressure and display the information on a numbered dial he can see. He then may, for example, be instructed to try to lower his blood pressure. He may shift his body position, try to relax, or think of a pleasant scene. If any action he takes lowers his blood pressure a detectable amount, he immediately learns of it so that he can continue to do whatever it was that helped to bring the dial reading down. That process makes for very efficient learning. In effect, it lets the reinforcer of signs of progress be immediately and continuously available for each effective effort. These procedures have been used to influence a person's self-control over a variety of body processes, such as blood pressure (Shapiro, Tursky, and Schwartz, 1970), brain-wave activity (Nowlis and Kamiya, 1970), and motor skills (Robb, 1968).

A number of direct treatment programs are based on biofeedback methods. For example, muscle tension pain may be reduced by training the person to relax certain muscle sets. This may be accomplished by attaching surface electrodes from an electromyograph to the site of muscle tension or muscle spasms. The amount of electrical activity (tension level) of the muscles then is portrayed in any of several ways, such as on a dial. The patient then may be able to try different procedures to relax himself. Given the continuous and precise information about the effectiveness of each method, he or she often quickly can find a way to bring down the tension level.

Developments with biofeedback methods have only begun. Within the next few years we can expect that many kinds of chronic conditions will lend themselves to modification or treatment with these techniques.

SUPPLEMENTAL READINGS

Brief and clear presentations of the principles of behavior analysis may also be found in a number of other sources. Four that we recommend particularly are: (1) Michael and Meyerson (1962): this article gives a brief and very lucid statement of the major principles of behavior analysis methods; (2) Patterson and Gullion (1968): this brief book is a programmed text designed to teach parents how to use behavior analysis methods in child rearing; it is very well done; (3) Holland and Skinner (1961): this is another programmed text that is very effectively done; (4) Reese (1966): this short book is a condensation of the principles of behavior analysis; it also describes experimental studies that provide part of the empirical basis for the methods. In addition to these four sources, there is a professional journal dedicated to the application of behavior analysis methods to human problems: *Journal of Applied Behavior Analysis,* published by the Society for the Experimental Analysis of Behavior, Lawrence, Kansas. Each issue of that quarterly journal contains many descriptions of applications of behavior analysis methods to a variety of human problems.

The extra readings cited here are not meant to be a complete list. We have chosen to mention sources that we are familiar with and that we feel will provide clear information pertinent to the needs of the health care professional who wishes to learn more about how he or she can use behavior analysis methods to help patients. The publications that would be useful in this regard are far too numerous to permit a comprehensive listing.

REFERENCES

American Nurses' Association: Guidelines for review of nursing care at the local level, Office of Professional Standards Review and Bureau of Quality Assurance Health Services Administration, Department of Health, Education and Welfare, 1967.

Ayllon, T., and Michael, J.: The psychiatric nurse as a behavioral engineer, Journal of the Experimental Analysis of Behavior 2:323-334, 1959.

Baer, D. M., and Wolf, M. M.: The entry into natural communities of reinforcement, Washington, D. C., 1967, American Psychological Association (mimeographed).

Berni, R.: The Berni nursing audit initiation tool, Seattle, Washington State Health Facilities Association, 1972 (mimeographed).

Berni, R., Dressler, J., and Baxter, J.: Reinforcing behavior, The American Journal of Nursing 71:2180-2183, November 1971.

Berni, R., and Readey, H.: Problem-oriented medical record implementation, St. Louis, 1974, The C. V. Mosby Co.

Bloom, J., Dressler, J., Kenny, M., and others: Problem-oriented charting, The American Journal of Nursing 71:2144-2148, November 1971.

Bushell, D., and Jacobson, J.: The simultaneous rehabilitation of mothers and their children in a working model for psychologists in rehabilitation. Symposium presented at Division 22, American Psychological Association, San Francisco, August 1968 (abstract, mimeographed).

Dinsdale, S. M., and others: The problem-oriented medical chart, The Archives of Physical Medicine Rehabilitation 51:488-492, August 1970.

Eisenberg, M., and Rustad, L.: Sex and the spinal cord injured: some questions and answers, 1975, ed. 2, Cleveland, Veterans Administration Hospital.

Fordyce, W., Fowler, R., Lehmann, J., and DeLateur, B.: Some implications of learning in problems of chronic pain, Journal of Chronic Diseases 21:179-190, 1968.

158

Fordyce, W., Fowler, R., Lehmann, J., Delateur, B., Sand, P., and Trieschmann, R.: Operant conditioning in the treatment of chronic pain, Arch. Phys. Med. Rehabil. **54:**399-408, September 1973.

Fordyce, W.: Behavioral methods for control of chronic pain and illness, St. Louis, 1976, The C. V. Mosby Co.

Fowler, R., Fordyce, W., and Berni, R.: Operant conditioning in chronic illness, The American Journal of Nursing **69:**1226-1228, June 1969.

Halpern, D., and Kottke, F.: Training of control of head posture in children with cerebral palsy, Developmental Medicine and Child Neurology **10:**249, 1968.

Holland, J. G., and Skinner, B. F.: The analysis of behavior, New York, 1961, McGraw-Hill Book Co.

Johnson, M., Davis, M. D., and Bilitch, M. J.: Problem-solving in nursing practice, Dubuque, 1970, William C. Brown Co.

Krusen, F., Kottke, F., and Ellwood, P.: Handbook of Physical Medicine and Rehabilitation, Philadelphia, 1971, W. B. Saunders Co.

Lindsley, O.: Geriatric behavioral prosthetics. In Kastenbaum, R., editor: New thoughts on old age, New York, 1964, Springer Publishing Co., pp. 41-60.

Marriner, A.: The nursing process, a scientific approach to nursing care, St. Louis, 1975, The C. V. Mosby Co.

Masters, W., and Johnson, V.: Human sexual response, Boston, 1966, Little, Brown and Co.

Michael, J., and Meyerson, L.: A behavioral approach to counseling and guidance, Harvard Educational Review **62:**382-402, Fall 1962.

Nowlis, D., and Kamiya, J.: The control of electroencephalographia alpha rhythms through auditory feedback and the associated mental activity, Psychophysiology **5:**476-484, January 1970.

Patterson, G. R.: Families: Applications of social learning to family life, Champaign, Ill., 1971, Research Press.

Patterson, G., and Gullion, M.: Living with children, Champaign, Ill., 1968, Research Press.

Premack, D.: Toward empirical behavior laws, I. Positive reinforcement, Psychology Review **66:**219-233, 1959.

Reese, E. P.: The analysis of human operant behavior, Dubuque, 1966, William C. Brown Co.

Rehabilitation publications and visual aids, Minneapolis, 1968, The American Rehabilitation Foundation.

Robb, J.: Feedback and skill learning, Research Quarterly **39:**175-184, March 1968.

Sand, P., and Berni, R.: A short term incentive contract: application patient care in nursing homes, The American Journal of Nursing, **74**(3):475-477, March 1974.

Shapiro, D., Tursky, B., and Schwartz, G.: Control of blood pressure in man by operant conditioning, Circulation Research **26** and **27** (Suppl. 1), July 1970.

Shelton, J. L., and Ackerman, J. M.: Homework in counseling and psychotherapy, Springfield, Ill., 1974, Charles C Thomas, Publisher.

Skinner, B. F.: Science and human behavior, New York, 1953, The Macmillan Co.

Tucker, S. M., and others: Patient care standards, St. Louis, 1975, The C. V. Mosby Co.

Wahler, R.: Oppositional children: a quest for parental reinforcement control, Journal of Applied Behavior Analysis **2:**159-170, 1969.

Weed, L. L.: Medical records, medical education and patient care, Cleveland, 1970, The Press of Case Western Reserve University.

Wenrich, W. W.: A primer of behavior modification, Belmont, 1970, Brooks/ Cole Publishing Co.

Zeilberger, J., Sampen, S., and Sloane, H.: Modification of a child's problem behaviors in the home with the mother as therapist, Journal of Applied Behavior Analysis **1:**47-53, 1968.

S